Echocardiography

and Cardiovascular Function:

Tools for the Next Decade

M.LeWinter. H. Suga and M.W. Watkins (eds.): *Cardiac Energetics: From Emax to Pressure-volume Area.* 1995   ISBN 0-7923-3721-2
R.J. Siegel (ed.): *Ultrasound Angioplasty.* 1995 ISBN 0-7923-3722-0
D.M. Yellon and G.J. Gross (eds.): *Myocardial Protection and the Katp Channel.* 1995   ISBN 0-7923-3791-3
A.V.G. Bruschke. J.H.C. Reiber. K.I. Lie and H.J.J. Wellens (eds.): *Lipid Lowering Therapy and Progression of Coronary Atherosclerosis.* 1996
                ISBN 0-7923-3807-3
A.S.A. Abd-Elfattah and A.S. Wechsler (eds.): *Purines and Myocardial Protection.* 1995   ISBN 0-7923-3831-6
M. Morad, S. Ebashi, W. Trautwein and Y. Kurachi (eds.): *Molecular Physiology and Pharmacology of Cardiac Ion Channels and Transporters.* 1996
                ISBN 0-7923-3913-4
A.M. Oto (ed.): *Practice and Progress in Cardiac Pacing and Electrophysiology.* 1996   ISBN 0-7923-3950-9
W.H. Birkenhager (ed.): *Practical Management of Hypertension. Second Edition.* 1996   ISBN 0-7923-3952-5
J.C. Chatham, J.R. Forder and J.H. McNeill(eds.):*The Heart In Diabetes.* 1996   ISBN 0-7923-4052-3
M. Kroll, M. Lehmann (eds.): *Implantable Cardioverter Defibrillator Therapy: The Engineering-Clinical Interface* 1996   ISBN 0-7923-4300-X
Lloyd Klein (ed.): *Coronary Stenosis Morphology: Analysis and Implication* 1996   ISBN 0-7923-9867-X
Julio E. Perez, Roberto M. Lang, (eds.): *Echocardiography and Cardiovascular Function: Tools for the Next Decade* 1996   ISBN 0-7923-9884-X

Echocardiography
and Cardiovascular Function:
Tools for the Next Decade

Editors:

Julio E. Pérez M.D.
Washington University
School of Medicine

Roberto M. Lang, M.D.
University of Chicago
School of Medicine

Associate Editor:

Victor Mor-Avi, Ph.D.
University of Chicago
School of Medicine

KLUWER ACADEMIC PUBLISHERS
Dordrecht / Boston / London

DISTRIBUTORS
For North America:
Kluwer Academic Publishers
101 Philip Drive
Norwell, Massachusetts 02061 USA
For all other countries:
Kluwer Academic Publishers Group
Distribution Centre
Post Office Box 322
3300 AH Dordrecht, THE NETHERLANDS
Library of Congress Cataloging-in-Publication Data

Echocardiography and cardiovascular function: tools for the next decade/editors, Julio E. Pérez, Roberto M. Lang:; associate editor, Victor Mor-Avi.
        p.   cm. -- (Developments in cardiovasculr medicine)
  Includes index.
  ISBN 0-7923-9884-X (alk. paper)
  1. Echocardiography. I. Pérez, Julio E.   II. Lang, Roberto M.
  III. Mor-Avi, Victor. IV. Series.
    [DNLM: 1. Echocardiography--methods. 2. Echocardiography--
    -instrumentation. 3. Heart Ventricle--ultrasonography. W1
    DE997VME 1997 / WG 141.5.E2 E1751 1997]
    RC683.5.U5E2434 1997
    616.1'207543--dc21
    DNLM/DLC
    for Library of Congress   97-4338
                                                                        CIP

Copyright 1997 by Kluwer Academic Publishers

Printed on acid-free paper.

Printed in the United States of America

Contents

Contributors

Amy C. Bales, M.D.
Assistant Professor of Medicine,
University of Chicago Medical Center, Chicago, Illinois

Chris M. Baumann, R.D.C.S.
Cardiac Sonographer, Echocardiography Laboratory,
Barnes and Jewish Hospitals, St. Louis, Missouri

James E. Bednarz, B.S., R.D.C.S.
Cardiac Sonographer, Noninvasive Cardiac Imaging Laboratory,
University of Chicago Medical Center, Chicago, Illinois

Sandra C. Gan, M.D.
Cardiologist, Minor and James Group
Seattle, Washington

John Gorcsan III, M.D.
Associate Professor of Medicine, Director of Echocardiography,
University of Pittsburgh Medical Center, Pittsburgh, Pennsylvania

Thomas R. Kimball, M.D.
Associate Professor of Pediatrics, Director of Cardiac Noninvasive
Imaging and Physiology Research Laboratory,
Children's Hospital Medical Center, Cincinnati, Ohio

Roberto M. Lang, M.D.
Professor of Medicine,
Director of Noninvasive Cardiac Imaging Laboratory,
University of Chicago Medical Center, Chicago, Illinois

Aleksandra Lange, M.D.
Western General Hospital, Edingburgh, Scotland, United Kingdom

Norma McDicken, M.D.
Professor of Medical Physics,
Western General Hospital, Edingburgh, Scotland, United Kingdom

Victor Mor-Avi, Ph.D.
Assistant Professor,
Research Associate, Noninvasive Cardiac Imaging Laboratory,
University of Chicago Medical Center, Chicago, Illinois

Przamyslaw Palka, M.D.
Western General Hospital, Edingburgh, Scotland, United Kingdom

Julio E. Pérez, M.D.
Professor of Medicine, Director of Echocardiography,
Washington University School of Medicine, St. Louis, Missouri

Richard L. Popp, M.D.
Professor of Medicine, Senior Associate Dean for Academic Affairs,
Stanford University Medical Center, Stanford, California

David Prater, M.A.
Engineer Scientist,
Hewlett Packard Company, Andover, Massachusetts

Sanjeev G. Shroff, Ph.D.
Professor of Medicine,
University of Chicago Medical Center, Chicago, Illinois

Kirk T. Spencer, M.D.
Assistant Professor of Medicine,
Associate Director of Noninvasive Cardiac Imaging Laboratory,
University of Chicago Medical Center, Chicago, Illinois

George R. Sutherland, M.D.
Senior Lecturer in Cardiology,
Western General Hospital, Edingburgh, Scotland, United Kingdom

Philippe Vignon, M.D.
Assistant Professor of Medicine,
Intensive Care Unit, University Hospital Dupuytren, Limoges, France

Alan D. Waggoner, M.H.S, R.D.M.S.
Chief Cardiac Sonographer, Barnes and Jewish Hospitals,
Research Instructor, Washington University, St. Louis, Missouri

Preface

For over a quarter of a century, echocardiography has made an unparalleled contribution to clinical cardiology as a major tool for real time imaging of cardiac dynamics. Echocardiography is widely used to assess cardiac function, and provides noninvasive information which is invaluable for the diagnosis of various disease states. In spite of its numerous advantages, in the clinical arena, echocardiography has remained mostly qualitative and subjective. However, continued progress in our understanding of the interactions between ultrasound and tissue characteristics have brought about several new developments, which allow quantitative analysis of ultrasound data. These exciting new techniques provide objective insight into important physiologic information hidden within ultrasound images, which is beyond the abilities of the human eye.

Among these new developments are endocardial boundary detection (frequently referred to as Acoustic Quantification), Color Kinesis and Doppler myocardial imaging, which have recently received considerable attention in the echocardiographic community. These techniques provide a more objective, robust and convenient evaluation of cardiac and vascular dynamics, that embraces multiple clinical applications. Over the past few years, these advances in cardiac ultrasound imaging have provided the opportunity for several groups of investigators worldwide to explore the applications of these novel techniques in various pathologies, and proved their clinical usefulness.

The purpose of this book is to provide the readers with the background necessary to understand and successfully utilize these methodologies. The following chapters summarize in detail the studies that have validated these techniques thus far, and discuss their future clinical applications. The results of this broad research effort more than suggest that, in the next decade, these new tools will become part of our routine clinical practice and bring more valuable objective information into clinical cardiology.

Acknowledgements

The editors and the authors wish to thank the cardiac sonographers with whom we have had the privilege of working throughout the years. Without their daily pursuit of quality, hard work and desire to continuously learn, this book would not have been completed.

We also owe a great debt to our colleagues who have collaborated with us closely. In particular, wish to acknowledge the invaluable help of Drs. Sanjeev Shroff, Kirk T. Spencer, Daniel Krauss, Victor G. Davila-Roman, Benico Barzilai and James G. Miller, who have been a pillar of outstanding scholarship and friendship to us.

We would also like to thank Dr. Jeffrey M. Leiden and Dr. Michael Cain, who have provided us with a positive and encouraging academic environment at the University of Chicago Medical Center and Washington University School of Medicine, respectively.

In addition, we want to express our gratitude to Debbie Taylor, Donna Barrett and Renata Bergunder for their expert secretarial assistance.

Finally, we would like to acknowledge our colleagues at the Imaging Systems Division of Hewlett Packard Company in Andover Massachusetts for their vision, ingenuity, extraordinary hard work and strong support.

1 The Fundamentals of Acoustic Quantification and Color Kinesis Technology

David Prater

Echocardiography is a very popular and useful tool for evaluating cardiac size and function. Its ability to produce real time two dimensional images allows for rapid visualization of the beating heart. To exploit this capability, both the sonographer and the cardiologist interpreting the ultrasound images require extensive training. Performing a proper ultrasound examination requires that the sonographer be knowledgeable on the correct placement of the transducer on the chest in order to obtain the desired views, optimal positioning of the patient in order to obtain the best images, and the techniques for adjusting the ultrasound system for the highest image quality. Evaluating the ultrasound images is an art that can literally take years to learn. One aspect which is particularly difficult to master is the evaluation of cardiac function. This particular information is usually judged qualitatively because, to date, it has been difficult and time consuming to produce automated quantitative measurements of cardiac function. Numerical values of cardiac chamber dimensions traditionally could only be obtained by manually tracing the contours of the cardiac chambers.

Numerous attempts have been made to assist the operator in this tracing task. The most popular approaches employed during the 1980's were based on edge detection algorithms [1-3], which attempted to locate transition zones in the gray scale image. These zones of transition are then assumed to represent "true" boundaries that exist because of differences in acoustic properties between different materials (*i.e.* blood vs. tissue). When applied to ultrasound images, these approaches have numerous limitations. The first issue concerns the speckle, manifested as the somewhat grainy pattern of the ultrasound images [4]. An edge detection algorithm may erroneously locate transitions within this grainy pattern, which do not constitute true boundaries between materials but simply fluctuations in intensity due to secondary reflections of ultrasound. A second limitation with edge detection is that the actual boundaries between materials may occur in multiple directions. In order to find these boundaries, every possible direction must be evaluated from every location within the image, which is a computationally expensive task.

As an alternative to traditional edge detection, the image can first be partitioned into different classes of materials [5]. The boundary is defined as the region where the materials with different acoustic properties meet. In the case of an ultrasound image, it can be partitioned into the blood-filled chamber and the surrounding tissue. The endocardial border is at the blood-tissue interface. Locating the boundary in this manner sufficiently simplifies the problem and accomplishes the task while an examination is being performed.

The approach employed by Acoustic Quantification (AQ - Hewlett Packard, Andover, MA) to partition the image into blood and tissue is based primarily on comparing the intensity of the received ultrasound signal against a pre-set threshold. Signals that are more intense than the threshold are classified as tissue and signals that are less intense are classified as blood. This rather simple classification technique is effective because the backscatter coefficient, or the ratio of reflected power to incident power, of myocardial tissue is considerably greater than that of blood. If a region of blood and a region of tissue are both insonified with the same amount of incident power, the tissue will backscatter a great deal more power than the blood.

For the classification approach to work, all regions composed of a similar material must produce approximately the same received signal intensity. Numerous aspects of traditional ultrasound imaging make this difficult to achieve. First, as an ultrasound wave propagates in the body, it attenuates. This attenuation affects both the forward propagating transmit pulse and the energy reflected back toward the transducer. Because of this attenuation, signals received from regions deeper into the body are less intense than signals received from closer structures. Second, the fixed transmit focus causes the intensity of the transmitted pulse to vary as a function of depth within the body. Thirdly, as the ultrasound beam is steered to produce the sector image used for cardiac imaging, the intensity of the received signal varies. This is due to the effective transducer aperture being smaller when the beam is steered to the side of the image than when the beam is steered towards the center of the image. Variation in beam intensity as a function of steering angle can also be affected by anatomical constraints such as the relative location of the ribs in the case of transthoracic echocardiography.

In order to compensate for these changes in received signal intensity which are unrelated to the material scattering properties, the sonographer has at his or her disposal a series of gain controls. These include an overall transmit gain, the time gain compensation (TGC) and the lateral gain compensation (LGC) controls (see Chapters 2 and 3). The overall transmit gain control allows the received signal intensity of the entire image to be adjusted to compensate for contact of the transducer with the chest wall and the attenuation that occurs through the chest wall. Compensation for changes in signal intensity as a function of depth are handled by the TGC controls while the LGC controls correct for changes in signal intensity as a function of beam steering angle.

The sonographer's adjustment of the gain controls has a significant impact on the quality of the ultrasound image. The success of an AQ study also depends on the operator to appropriately adjust the gain controls. To correctly classify all regions as either tissue or blood, the gain controls must be adjusted so that all regions of similar material exhibit similar intensities. This is basically the same adjustment the user would do to obtain high quality ultrasound image. The user then activates the AQ border display which will indicate with an "orange" border where it detects the interfaces between the blood pools and the surrounding tissue. If all the tissue regions have intensities above the AQ threshold and all blood regions have intensities below the threshold, then the border will be positioned directly over the endocardial border in every frame of the image. If the border is not positioned correctly, then the user will need to modify the gain controls to adjust the intensities of the blood and tissue regions using the position of the "orange" border as a guide.

Many of the publications of clinical and laboratory animal studies employing AQ have noted that the AQ processing is performed on the "raw RF" signal. This "raw RF" or unprocessed radiofrequency signal is the output of the beam forming electronics, including all TGC and LGC controls, but not including the video processing of the compression and post-processing controls. These video processing controls allow the user to adjust the gray scale appearance of the image. In the designing of the system it was considered desirable to allow the operator to adjust the image using these controls without influencing the blood/tissue classification. Therefore the AQ processing is performed utilizing this unprocessed radiofrequency signal rather than the more processed video signal.

The binary image which results from the classification of regions of the image into blood and tissue can be used directly to quantify the area of the blood pool. Typically, the operator is not interested in the blood area of the entire image but rather the blood area of a particular chamber. A user definable region of interest allows the selection of a specific chamber. Due to the irregular geometry of cardiac chambers in various pathologies, this region of interest needs to be of arbitrary shape. AQ offers two techniques to the operator for outlining the region of interest. The first is to trace the region of interest using the system's trackball. This tracing should include the entire chamber of interest and exclude other chambers. Since the system has identified each region of the image as either blood or tissue, the traced region of interest can include as much tissue as desired. When calculating the blood pool area within the region of interest the system will ignore the included tissue.

While this approach of tracing the region of interest may result in an arbitrarily shaped region, this method is very tedious. For that reason, a second method is available for the operator to define the region of interest. Using two or three points, a stylized region of interest in the shape of either a circle or a half ellipsoid can be positioned over the cardiac chamber blood pool area of interest. Once located, the system will analyze the signals samples within these stylized shapes and identify which are blood and which are tissue.

Once the region of interest has been positioned in the image, the system will determine the blood area within the region in every acoustic frame. Typically, area values will be generated at a rate of approximately 30 Hz [6]. These discrete values can be used to generate a continuous signal by interpolation. Mathematical curves are fitted to the discrete area values. These curves are connected to form a continuous waveform. For AQ, the mathematical curves used for interpolation are multi-point polynomials. The use of these particular curves requires that both the waveform and its time derivative are continuous.

Ultrasound images are actually two dimensional slices of three dimensional structures (*i.e.* muscle or blood pool chambers). Therefore, the AQ blood/tissue classification allows the calculation of the blood pool area of a chosen region of the image which is actually a slice through a three dimensional blood volume. The area value can then be extrapolated to estimate the three dimensional volume of the chamber by making a number of different geometric assumptions. Two different methods are provided in AQ for carrying out this extrapolation using the echocardiographic apical views. These methods are the method of summation of disks (MOD, Simpson's rule) and the area-length method.

For the MOD technique (Figure 1.1,A), the detected blood region is rotated around an axis to form an irregular circularly symmetric volume. This is accomplished by subdividing the region of interest into twenty parallel slices which are perpendicular to the axis around which the blood region is to be rotated. As each of these slices is rotated around the axis, they form a short cylinder the diameter of which is the width of blood pool area within the slice. The estimated volume of the three dimensional chamber is the sum of the volumes of the cylinders from each slice. The main geometric assumption for this technique is that the three dimensional structure can be accurately reproduced by simply rotating the area around the long axis.

The area-length method assumes that the blood area is a half-ellipse, and represents a slice through a half-ellipsoid (Figure 1.1,B). This volume of the half-ellipsoid can be calculated from its area and length. There are more assumptions inherent to the shape of the three dimensional structure when using the area-length method than by the MOD method and therefore, this method is not as accurate for quantification of volume of chambers whose shape differs significantly from half-ellipsoid. Both volume estimation methods require the use of apical views as these are the only views that permit the entire long axis of the heart to be imaged.

These volume estimation techniques assume that the two dimensional slice passes directly through the central axis of the three dimensional volume. In the practice of echocardiography it is very common to inadvertently foreshorten the true length of the apical images. Rather than placing the two dimensional slice directly through the central axis of the left ventricular volume, a slice is angled through the volume. This shortens the true major axis of the left ventricle and leads to underestimation of the true cavity volume.

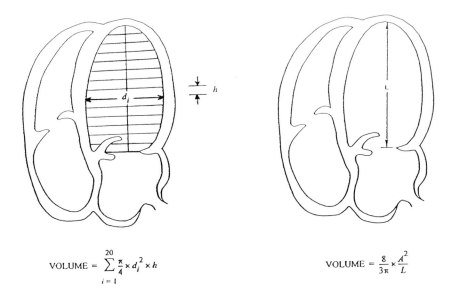

$$\text{VOLUME} = \sum_{i=1}^{20} \frac{\pi}{4} \times d_i^2 \times h$$

$$\text{VOLUME} = \frac{8}{3\pi} \times \frac{A^2}{L}$$

Figure 1.1. Two volume computation methods are provided by AQ: method of disks (MOD, left), and area-length method (right).

The area and volume waveforms produced by AQ are a valuable aid in the evaluation of global cardiac function on-line. Many useful measurements can be obtained from these waveforms, and the AQ system generates several of these automatically. These include the chambers' end-diastolic volume, end-systolic volume, ejection fraction, peak filling rate, peak ejection rate and time to peak filling rate. Every cardiac cycle these values are measured from the waveforms and displayed as numeric readouts next to the waveform display. An ECG R-wave detector is used to identify the start of each cardiac cycle, and it is critical that this detector identifies every R-wave rather than other portions of the ECG as R-waves. If the system erroneously selects a T-wave as an R-wave, then the normal R-R interval would be divided into two intervals, R-T and T-R. This would have an adverse effect on the calculation of the values measured from the waveforms since these values are measured at certain times within the R-R interval. The operator can avoid this error by correctly positioning the three leads of the ECG monitor. Placing the leads so that the voltage of the R-waves exceeds that of the T-wave will make it easier for the system to correctly identify R-waves and reject the T-waves.

Because in coronary artery disease, cardiac dysfunction first manifests itself in a regional rather than global manner, an enhancement has been recently added to AQ to assist in the detection of these abnormalities. This enhancement has been named Color Kinesis to highlight its ability to display the temporal and spatial patterns of cardiac chamber endocardial motion (see Chapters 10 and 11). The basis of Color Kinesis is the same blood/tissue classification of AQ. However, rather than accumulating the blood pool area for each acoustic time frame as in the case of AQ, Color Kinesis detects changes in the classification status for each pixel of each acoustic frame. When a pixel changes classification from one acoustic frame to the next, this change is assumed to represent motion. Under most conditions, this is a reasonable assumption, since the properties of the blood and the tissue change very littler (if at all) over the cardiac cycle. The change in classification of a pixel is usually due to endocardial wall motion as the cardiac chamber either contracts or expands. For example, a pixel located within the left ventricle near the endocardial border will be a blood pixel at the end of diastole. As systole proceeds and the heart contracts, the myocardium will thicken and the endocardial border will move inward. As it does, the pixel that was classified as blood, becomes tissue.

Color Kinesis operates as a display sequence, *i.e.* there is one sequence per cardiac cycle (Figure 1.2). The sequence begins at a specified start time and runs for a specified duration. Beginning at the start time, each pixel is exmined in each consecutive acoustic frame, and the first time that it undergoes a transition, it is assigned a color. Different color hues are used to mark pixels which change classification at different times within the display sequence. At the end of the display sequence, all pixels which have changed classification will have been designated with the color representing the time of their transition (from tissue to blood or blood to tissue, depending on the outward expansion or inward contraction phase of the heart). The resultant color image will appear as a series of irregularly shaped colored concentric rings. The width of the color pattern for each section of the concentric ring structure shows the amount of wall motion for that section in each frame of the image (typically 33 ms), and the width of each individual color shows the temporal pattern of the motion. On the acoustic frame following the end of the display sequence, all colors are removed from the image in preparation for the next display sequence during the following cardiac cycle. Thus, Color Kinesis allows a frame-by-frame visualization of the temporal and spatial pattern of endocardial motion.

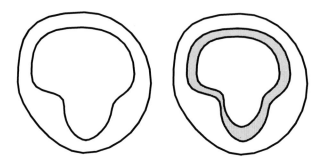

Figure 1.2. Similar to AQ, Color Kinesis is based on a frame-by-frame blood/tissue pixel classification. Pixels which change from blood to tissue are assumed to have done so due to contractile endocardial motion. This figure shows scematically how pixels that changed from blood to tissue from end-diastolic frame (left) to first frame of systole (right) are color-encoded using a color overlay superimposed on the gray scale image. A different color is used for each frame of systole. The overlay colors accumulate from frame to frame, producing a display of the time-motion history of endocardial motion from end-diastole to end-systole.

Endocardial motion can be broadly separated into two phases, a contraction phase and an expansion phase. Color Kinesis has separate modes, contract and expand, to match these different phases. Since Color Kinesis is not restricted to motion of the left ventricle, it was deemed more general to use the terms contract and expand rather than systole and diastole. For both the contract and expand modes, it is necessary to specify when the Color Kinesis display sequence should start, and its total duration. A third mode exists which is best suited for evaluation of the left ventricle. In this mode, called systole, the operator does not need to specify the start time and the duration of display sequence, as these are determined automatically by the system. Display sequence always starts with the R-wave, and its duration is determined based on the prevailing heart rate of the patient at the time of the examination.

In the contract mode, Color Kinesis uses different colors to mark those pixels which change from blood to tissue at different times within the contraction phase. Some pixels may not change from blood to tissue but rather from tissue to blood during this contracting phase. In this case this type of endocardial motion would represent a "paradoxical" motion pattern. To highlight these pixels, Color Kinesis encodes them with a read color, called the "dyskinesis color". For the expand mode, pixels changing from tissue to blood are marked with the time dependent colors, and pixels which change from blood to tissue are marked with the dyskinesis color.

Once a pixel is assigned a color, that color remains until all colors are removed at the end of the display sequence. The pixels are assigned colors based on their first change of classification. During a display sequence, a pixel may change from tissue to blood in the first frame and then change from blood to tissue in subsequent frames. If Color Kinesis is in the contract mode when this occurs, the pixel will be assigned the dyskinesis color, since the first transition of tissue to blood represents this "paradoxical", albeit physiologic, motion in the contract mode.

In summary, the blood/tissue pixel classification applied to echocardio-graphic images has been proven helpful in evaluating global cardiac performance in real time. Color Kinesis has extended this capability to facilitate the evaluation of regional function. Its unique display format allows both the spatial and temporal patterns of regional endocardial motion to be visualized. There is a great deal of information which can be extracted from the AQ waveforms and the Color Kinesis display. In the following chapters, the clinical applications of acoustic quantification and Color Kinesis are described in detail.

References

1. Collins SM, Skorton DJ, Geiser EA, Nichols JA, Conetta DA, Pandian NG, Kerber RE: Computer-assisted edge detection in two-dimensional echocardiography: Comparison with anatomical data. *Am J Cardiol* 1984;53:1380-1387.
2. Geiser EA, Oliver LH, Gardin J, Kerber RE, Parisi AF, Reichek N, Werner JA, Weyman AE: Clinical validation of an edge detection algorithm for two-dimensional echocardiographic short-axis images. *J Am Soc Echocardiogr* 1988;1:410-421.
3. Jenkins JM: Computer processing of echocardiographic images for automated edge detection of left ventricular boundaries. *IEEE Transac Computers Cardiol*, 1981;391-394.
4. Melton HE, Collins SM, Skorton DJ: Automatic real-time endocardial edge detection in two-dimensional echocardiography. *Ultrasonic Imaging* 1983;5:300-307.
5. Abbott JG, Thurstone FL: Acoustic speckle theory and experimental analysis. *Ultrasonic Imaging* 1979;1:303-324.
6. Hui WKK, Gibson DG: The dynamics of rapid left ventricular filling in man. *Adv Cardiol* 1985;32:7-35.

2 How to Perform an Acoustic Quantification Study: Technical Factors Influencing Study Quality and Pitfalls to Avoid

James E. Bednarz, Chris M. Baumann
and Roberto M. Lang

Acoustic Quantification (AQ) is an image processing border detection system (Hewlett-Packard Sonos 1500 and 2500, Andover, MA) that provides on-line, beat-to-beat values for left ventricular (LV) cavity area and volume. These measurements can then be used to calculate load-dependent parameters of systolic performance such as ejection fraction and stroke volume in real-time. In addition, it is possible to generate load-independent parameters of systolic performance such as end-systolic pressure-volume relations (see Chapters 6 and 9). By providing on-line estimations of clinically important but previously inaccessible physiologic parameters, AQ technology facilitates a quantitative assessment of hemodynamic responses to pharmacologic and surgical interventions. Although many studies have validated the use of AQ techniques, this boundary detection system, like other diagnostic ultrasound modalities, is highly operator dependent. This chapter will discuss the technical aspects of acquiring optimal AQ data and identify the potential pitfalls and limitations.

Acquisition of AQ Data

Overview

For every frame, AQ analyzes backscatter data along each scan line before it is processed into video data and designates each pixel as either tissue or blood (see Chapter 1). This tissue-blood designation is determined by comparing each pixel's backscatter value to fixed thresholds. The operator uses the *gain, time-gain compensation (TGC)*, and *lateral gain* controls (*LGC*) to adjust the pixel backscatter values by visually aligning the AQ border with the LV endocardial border. In the "blood" mode, all pixels designated as blood are assigned a red color, whereas in the "border" mode, only those pixels designated as representing an endocardial border are assigned a color. By drawing a region of interest encompassing the LV, a waveform of LV area versus time can be displayed in real-time representing the area of all pixels designated as blood within the region of interest. A volume waveform can be obtained from apical images by using geometric formulas based on single plane measurements. The AQ system can display:

1. waveforms of areas or volumes;
2. waveforms of the derivatives of these areas or volumes;
3. digital beat to beat values for:
   - end-diastolic area or volume;
   - end-systolic area or volume;
   - fractional area change (area) or ejection fraction (volume);
   - peak filling rate and peak ejection rate (derivatives);
   - time to peak filling rate.

Reliable determination of LV areas, volumes, and their derivatives using AQ depends upon numerous factors. These include accurate tracking of the LV endocardial borders, reproducible transducer positioning, and proper alignment of imaging planes to obtain the true long axis of the ventricle [1]. Two different geometric and mathematical models for the calculation of LV volume from a long-axis image have been incorporated into the ultrasound equipment (see Chapter 1). The method of discs (MOD) divides the ventricle into 20 circular discs and calculates the total LV volume by Simpson's rule. The area-length method uses the LV length and area acquired from an apical view to calculate volume [2]. Because LV volumes are derived by applying predetermined geometric models to LV area measurements, potential sources of inaccuracy include both measurement errors associated with LV area determinations and inappropriate geometric assumptions regarding the shape of the ventricle. The MOD assumes that each disc is circular and rotated around the LV long axis, whereas the area-length method assumes that the ventricle is an ellipsoid. Although these assumptions are not always valid, in almost all cases, the MOD formula should more accurately determine left ventricular volume because it is based on fewer geometric assumptions. The area-length formula was included because it is an accepted single plane standard for volume calculations. The most obvious reason to employ the area-length formula is when comparing an AQ volume calculation to another technique that also uses the area-length formula. Clinical and experimental studies have demonstrated that AQ-derived LV areas and volumes correlate well with both off-line, manual echocardiographic measurements as well as data obtained using imaging modalities such as magnetic resonance imaging, radionuclide ventriculography, and ultrafast computed tomography [3-12] (see Chapter 3).

Ultrasound System Setup

The ultrasonographer should adjust the video monitor settings, pre-processing and post-processing curves in order to optimally visualize the endocardial-blood interface. Before beginning the AQ study, the sonographer should adjust the monitor screen according to the examining room ambient light conditions. To properly adjust the monitor, both the brightness and contrast controls should be moved to their maximum levels. Carefully observing the gray levels scale bar on the right side of the image, the brightness control should be slowly turned counterclockwise to decrease the brightness until the operator can visually distinguish between the two darker gray levels on the gray scale bar. The darkest gray level indicator should just barely blend into the gray screen background. In the case of a black background, the darkest gray scale bar should just barely be distinguished from the black background. The contrast control should then be adjusted until screen typographical characters are clear. Once the monitor is properly adjusted, the actual boundary between endocardium and blood will be much easier to identify, without inadvertent use of the overall transmit gain control (which influences the blood pool cavity area measurement) for this purpose.

A smooth electrocardiographic signal with an upright R wave is necessary to trigger the digital AQ values. This is best accomplished by placing the white electrode (RA) over the patient's right shoulder, the black electrode (LA) over the patient's lower left chest, and the red electrode (LL) over the patient's left shoulder resulting in a large upright R wave to allow proper timing of the physiologic cavity area or volume.

Two-Dimensional Imaging

Acoustic Quantification relies on adequate definition of LV endocardial boundaries in order to accurately align the border. Accordingly, obtaining a two-dimensional image optimized for endocardial definition is a crucial step in performing a technically adequate AQ study. The AQ data can be acquired in the parasternal short-axis view and the apical two and four chamber views of the LV when these views demonstrate adequate endocardial visualization using transthoracic or transesophageal echocardiography. The imaging planes should consist of conventional and reproducible tomographic cuts to ensure meaningful comparisons with prior or subsequent studies.

The parasternal short-axis view should be obtained at the mid-papillary muscle level to avoid tracking of the mitral valve apparatus at any time during the acquisition period. The imaging plane is defined by observing both papillary muscles with the final imaging plane position obtained by alternatively angling and rotating the transducer to avoid an oblique imaging plane [13].

A technically adequate apical four-chamber view is obtained by placing the transducer directly over the anatomic cardiac apex and directing the ultrasound beam toward the base of the heart. The imaging plane is defined by obtaining the true LV apex and maximal excursion of both the mitral and tricuspid valves. Positioning the transducer at the point of maximal impulse is a good starting point, but adjustments in transducer positioning are usually necessary to avoid a foreshortened apical image. A foreshortened view is characterized by a blunt, flattened appearance of the apex indicating that the imaging plane does not pass through the true apex. In the case of foreshortening, the correct transducer position can be located by progressively imaging the LV in a short-axis view and repositioning it down the chest wall until the LV cavity obliterates at the apex. To obtain a technically adequate, non-foreshortened apical image, the sonographer should strive to obtain the maximal LV length and maximal excursion of both atrioventricular valves [13].

The apical two-chamber view is obtained from the same transducer position as the non-foreshortened apical four-chamber view. The transducer is rotated counterclockwise to completely exclude right ventricular structures and is then aligned parallel to the true long-axis of the LV by obtaining the maximal LV diameter at the base [13].

In patients with regional wall motion abnormalities, if a regional abnormality is present but not visualized in the chosen view, using only one imaging plane will overestimate the ejection fraction. Conversely, the ejection fraction will be underestimated if a discrete regional abnormality is visualized in the chosen plane while the remaining left ventricular segments contract vigorously. In the presence of regional abnormalities, a more accurate technique for determining an ejection fraction is to average the ejection fractions obtained in both apical four and two-chamber views.

Alignment of AQ Borders

After optimizing the two-dimensional image and activating the AQ borders, visual alignment of the AQ borders with the two-dimensional endocardial boundaries is performed using three types of gain controls: 1) the *transmit gain* control which adjusts the transmit and receive gain for the entire image, 2) the *lateral gain compensation* controls (LGC) which adjust the receive gain in eight adjacent sectors, and 3) the *time gain compensation* (TGC) controls which adjust the receive gain at eight different depths (Figure 2.1). The compression setting does not influence the calculation of the blood pool cavity area and can therefore be freely adjusted to assist in the visual recognition of the endocardial-blood interface.

The transmit or overall gain should be initially adjusted to ensure that the AQ borders track the endocardial border for as many LV segments as possible. This is best done by closely observing the location of the endocardium on the real-time conventional 2D image, then activating the boundary detection algorithm. By repeatedly engaging the border detection (on and off) several times, the operator can determine that each endocardial segment is tracking appropriately. The sonographer should carefully ascertain that true endocardium is detected as opposed to the mid-myocardial echoes, mitral valve structures, papillary muscle or chordae. Often, slight transducer angulation can correct this, incorporating small "islands" that appear to lie within the blood pool that would be incorrectly excluded as part of the true endocardial boundary. Similarly, noise artifact within the blood pool cavity should be minimized or eliminated with transducer angulation.

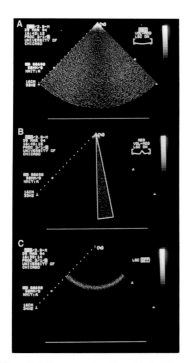

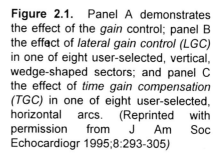

Figure 2.1. Panel A demonstrates the effect of the *gain* control; panel B the effect of *lateral gain control (LGC)* in one of eight user-selected, vertical, wedge-shaped sectors; and panel C the effect of *time gain compensation (TGC)* in one of eight user-selected, horizontal arcs. (Reprinted with permission from J Am Soc Echocardiogr 1995;8:293-305)

The *TGC* controls should initially be positioned at their mid-point to facilitate the adjustment of each control. These controls are useful to adjust AQ tracking at the apex and the level of the mitral valve annulus. The TGC controls should also be used to "white-out" the left atrial cavity area below the mitral annulus, which precludes the inclusion of the left atrium into the measurement of the volume or cavity area of the left ventricle which is being measured.

The *LGC* controls should initially be set at their minimum position with settings increased as required to optimize AQ border tracking. It is recommended that the operator adjust the right-side controls first by gradually increasing gain in small increments, working toward the left-side of the image until adequate gain is attained (see Chapter 3). The largest increase in lateral gain should occur at the far sides, in order to avoid unusual high gain in the middle of the image sector that may compromise the measurements. The *LGC* profile on the imaging screen graphically reflects the position of the *LGC* controls and should demonstrate a smooth, gradual variation in gain settings. When an individual *LGC* control is set too high, the corresponding sector becomes visibly brighter than the adjacent sectors; this may create a stationary "false wall" that impairs tracking of LV endocardial motion.

Alignment of the AQ borders with the endocardial boundaries can be performed using either of two basic approaches. Using the first approach, the sonographer initially adjusts the *gain* until the AQ borders track as much of the endocardial boundaries as possible. The *TGC* and *LGC* controls are then used to fine-tune the tracking in the areas that are not tracking accurately (Figure 2.2). The second technique is recommended for sonographers with less experience visualizing both AQ and endocardial borders simultaneously. To begin, the *gain* is increased until the AQ borders are located within the LV cavity. The AQ borders often become speckled or broken-up at high gain settings. The *TGC* and *LGC* controls are then adjusted to ensure that the AQ borders are centered within the cavity and are equidistant from the true endocardial boundaries for the entire LV. The *gain* is then decreased until the AQ borders "snap to" the two-dimensional endocardial boundaries (Figure 2.2). The final step for both techniques is to toggle the AQ borders on and off to verify accurate tracking of the endocardial boundary throughout the cardiac cycle.

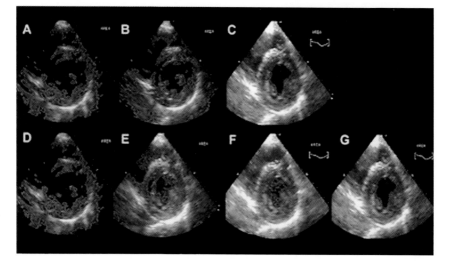

Figure 2.2. The methods used for aligning the AQ borders with the endocardial boundaries. Panels A and D show a parasternal short-axis view of the LV after optimizing image quality and activating the AQ mode. Method 1 (top) consists of adjusting the *gain* control to track as much of the LV as possible (B). Then, fine-tuning of the *TGC* and *LGC* controls is performed (C). Method 2 (bottom) initially uses high *gain* such that the AQ borders are within the LV cavity (E). The *TGC* and *LGC* controls are then used to align the AQ borders within the LV cavity so that they are equidistant from the endocardial boundaries (F). The *gain* is then decreased until the AQ borders "snap-to" the endocardial boundaries (G).

Selection of a Region of Interest

The AQ system will calculate areas or volumes for a specific region of interest (ROI) that the user may select. A ROI can be drawn either by manual tracing or by a semi-automatic drawing method (quick ROI) based on the positioning of two or three points using a trackball (Figure 2.3).

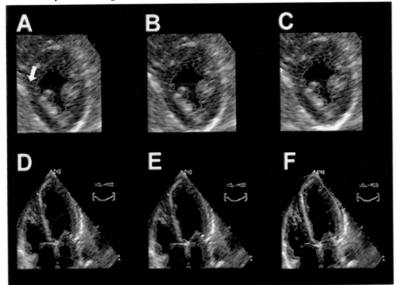

Figure 2.3. The upper panels illustrate the two-point method of designating a region of interest for a short-axis view of the LV. The lower panels show the three-point method for an apical-four chamber view of the LV.

The two-point quick ROI method is used for the parasternal short-axis view of the LV. This method uses two points to define the diameter of a circular region of interest. The three-point quick ROI uses two points at the mitral annulus and one point distal to the apex to define a hemi-ellipsoidal region of interest for apical four-chamber and two-chamber images of the LV. This approach is best for normally shaped LV cavities. To employ the three point method, the operator activates the ROI control, which displays the first cross-hair over the image. The first point should be placed at the left atrial side of the mitral annulus at end-diastole. A second marker is to be placed at the right side of the mitral annulus, and a third marker is placed at the cardiac apex just above the endocardium, so that all of the endocardial borders will be encompassed by the ROI. The lower portion of the ROI should be positioned across the plane of the mitral annulus. If the left ventricle is aneurysmal or crescent-shaped (non-ellipsoidal), it may be easier to employ the manual approach of drawing a ROI. This is performed by activating the ROI control, placing the point at the lower right side of the mitral annulus, and outlining the left ventricular cavity area just outside the endocardium. The auto-close option will complete the ROI by drawing a straight line through the mitral annulus, and final approval will set the ROI before proceeding with the measurements. Once approved, the ROI can be adjusted using the size and position controls with the trackball to ensure that: 1) the LV cavity remains within the ROI throughout the cardiac cycle, and 2) the right ventricle and left atrium do not move into the ROI at any time.

In the volume mode, the AQ software displays a long axis of the left ventricle which is then used for the MOD volume calculation. It is determined by the midpoint of the auto-close line and the point on the ROI line at the apex that is farthest from the mitral annulus. The operator can modify this automatic long axis if necessary. In addition, tracing of the ROI at the apex should be sufficiently close to the apical endocardium to maximize the number of volume slices when the volume is being calculated by the method of discs (Figure 2.4).

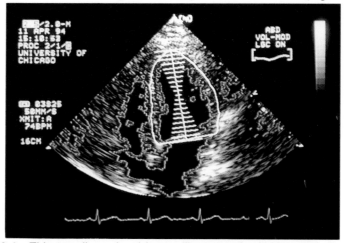

Figure 2.4. This two-dimensional image illustrates the LV long-axis line in an apical four-chamber view. The long-axis line is divided into twenty segments representing the twenty circular discs that the method of discs (MOD) formula uses to calculate LV volume. The MOD calculates the volume of each of the discs and then sums them to determine the total volume of the LV cavity. *(Reprinted with permission from J Am Soc Echocardiogr 1995;8:293-305)*

Displaying Waveforms

Options for the display of waveforms are selected by the user and include area or volume curves and/or their derivatives. Calibration values should be adjusted for maximum resolution. Current AQ software includes an automatic waveform calibration feature that employs a *rescale* button to automatically optimize the waveform size. When using earlier versions of the AQ software, the most efficient way to adjust the calibration is to first position the nadir of the curve at the bottom of the screen by adjusting the minimum scale value and secondly to increase the size of the waveform by increasing the scale increment value. Asking a cooperative patient to briefly suspend respiration for approximately five seconds can aid in obtaining optimal, consistent recordings of AQ waveforms by eliminating both the respiratory influence on LV chamber size (*i.e.* physiologic preload changes) as well as respiratory-induced artifact.

Current AQ software offers an averaging mode that displays a mean value with standard deviation for all digitally displayed measurements and indicates the number of beats used to calculate the means and standard deviations. Averaging techniques may be useful to overcome the beat-to-beat variability sometimes noted for individual patient data (Figure 2.5). The operator can modify the averaging parameters which include the number of beats, waveform variability based on minimum and maximum values, and heart rate variability.

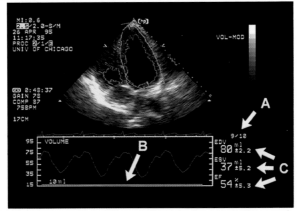

Figure 2.5. This frame of an AQ waveform in the averaging mode displays the number of beats averaged (beats that met the user-controlled criteria) versus the number of beats considered (arrow A), a blue line that indicates which waveforms have been included in the computation of the average values (arrow B), and also the standard deviation for each digital value (arrows C).

The sweep speed of the waveform can be adjusted. In the case of a clinical study to determine an ejection fraction, a frozen screen at a sweep speed of 25 mm/sec will display more beats than faster scrolling speeds and thus allow better visual assessment of the consistency of the waveforms in terms of maximum and minimum values and waveform shape. The frozen waveform screen can then be printed or videotaped. For research purposes, relaying the analog waveform output from the optional "dataport" on the ultrasound equipment directly into a computer is an efficient way to record AQ data.

Once optimal AQ waveforms have been obtained, system parameters including the region of interest, *gain*, *LGC*, *TGC*, *compress*, and *depth* settings can be saved into a "'preset" memory control called *gain save* for each of four conventional imaging views. Thus the saved system settings can be recalled as the images are repeatedly obtained, and AQ data can usually be re-acquired with only minor system adjustments. This is particularly useful to improve consistency when obtaining sequential AQ and CK data during pharmacological stress testing.

Recording AQ Data

Before recording AQ waveforms, the sonographer should quickly review: (1) the two dimensional image to verify that the AQ system is accurately tracking the endocardial border and that the ROI is properly placed, (2) the waveforms to verify that the maximum and minimum values are consistent and that the waveforms are smooth and similar in shape, and (3) the digital display of AQ values to verify that they are consistent with small standard deviations. When satisfied with the data quality, the sonographer should record the AQ data (during held end-expiration if necessary).

Learning to Perform AQ Studies

An ultrasonographer learning to perform AQ studies can divide an AQ study into three component parts, practice one until proficient, and then add the second component, and later the third portion; this stepwise approach may make the process more efficient. Initially the sonographer should select patients with clearly visualized endocardial borders by two-dimensional imaging and adjust the three types of gain in a methodical way such that the AQ signal tracks as accurately as possible. The second step should consist of adjusting the gain settings plus also drawing the region of interest. When proficient at these two skills, the final step would be to obtain waveforms in addition to setting gain levels and drawing the region of interest. Several studies have demonstrated that AQ studies are reproducible, can be performed accurately on 70% to 80% of all patients, and with experience should not significantly increase the duration of a clinical study [14-16] (see Chapter 3).

Sources of Error

The sonographer must be skilled and experienced with AQ to obtain high quality data consistently. A discussion of the most common technical pitfalls will shorten the learning process.

ECG

Digital AQ values are based on an ECG trigger; if the ECG is not present or noisy, the border and waveforms will appear on the screen but the numerical values will not. The ECG is as important for an AQ study as it is for a stress echo study.

Gain Settings

Proper gain settings are the most crucial aspect of performing a good quality AQ study. The transmit or total gain is too high if any border other than the apex is tracking within the left ventricular cavity. Borders that are tracking outside the endocardium and need increased gain can be manipulated using the LGC and/or TGC controls. Typically, the lateral wall of the left ventricle in an apical four-chamber view is the most difficult region to track accurately. In this case, the LGC should be increased gradually in the sectors corresponding to the lateral wall until the AQ borders accurately track the lateral wall endocardium. Too great an increase in the LGC creates a "false wall" which can be visualized as a bright, vertical band of echoes that impairs tracking of the endocardium during systole (Figure 2.6). In a small number of patients, two-dimensional image quality may be inadequate for accurate AQ tracking of endocardial boundaries.

Imaging Plane

If the patient has had a previous AQ study, it is essential to review these images to ensure that an identical imaging plane is used. There can be a significant variation in AQ data depending on the imaging plane. In addition, the plane must not foreshorten the LV apex, even at the expense of a poorly visualized apex. To illustrate the significance of a foreshortened left ventricular apex, Figure 2.7 demonstrates the differences for LV length, systolic and diastolic volumes, and ejection fraction for a foreshortened and a non-foreshortened apical imaging plane.

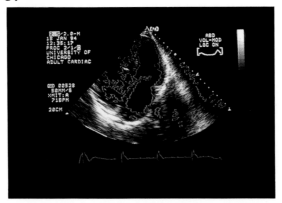

Figure 2.6. This example of a "false wall" created by too high an adjustment for an individual *LGC* control is identified by the sharp peak in the *LGC* profile and by the wedge of the 2D sector that appears visibly brighter than the remainder of the image. This "false wall" may impair AQ tracking of LV endocardial motion.

If regional wall motion abnormalities are present, the ejection fraction may vary depending on which apical view is used for the AQ study. Therefore, it is important that a complete two-dimensional examination is performed prior to the AQ study to assess regional function. As previously discussed, if regional abnormalities are present, the ejection fraction should be averaged from two apical views. If no regional wall motion abnormality is detected, an apical four-chamber view should provide a representative left ventricular ejection fraction.

Respiratory Variation

Respiratory variations in AQ waveforms are commonly observed, especially in dyspneic patients. There are two possible explanations for this variation:
1. In a normal heart, inspiration leads to a fall in intrathoracic pressure which in turn results in increased systemic venous return. As a consequence, right ventricular size increases, shifting the interventricular septum into the left ventricle, which in turn decreases left ventricular size. These respiratory variations in volume constitute real, physiologic changes.

2.   Respiration may also introduce variation into an AQ signal by altering the imaging plane, changing the position of the ROI, or even obscuring the LV.

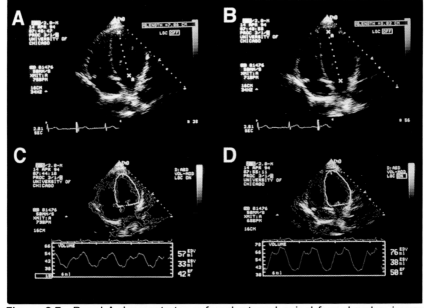

Figure 2.7. Panel A demonstrates a foreshortened apical four-chamber image as compared to a non-foreshortened view from the same patient in panel B. The end-diastolic left ventricular long-axis length for the foreshortened view is 7.06 cm, compared to a length of 8.02 cm for the non-foreshortened image. Panel C presents the AQ waveform associated with the foreshortened view in panel A, while panel D corresponds to the non-foreshortened image in panel B. The digital AQ values for end-diastolic volume, end-systolic volume, and ejection fraction are all significantly smaller for the foreshortened image compared to the values obtained for the non-foreshortened view. (*Reprinted with permission from J Am Soc Echocardiogr 1995;8:293-305*)

Figure 2.8 demonstrates the significant variations in AQ waveforms that may be noted with respiration. To limit this respiratory variation, it is important to record during held end-expiration or use the averaging feature.

Displacement of the ROI

During an AQ study, multiple factors may result in displacement of the heart relative to the ROI. Minimal patient or sonographer movement may alter the position of the image relative to the designated ROI. Similarly, respiration or excessive motion of the mitral annulus relative to the ROI may be problematic. The patient and sonographer should both be in comfortable positions, and AQ data should be recorded at end-expiration as necessary. Also, to emphasize a previous point, it is important to perform the AQ study quickly, to check the two-dimensional echocardiographic image for proper tracking and ROI placement, and to verify that the waveforms and the digital display are consistent immediately before recording.

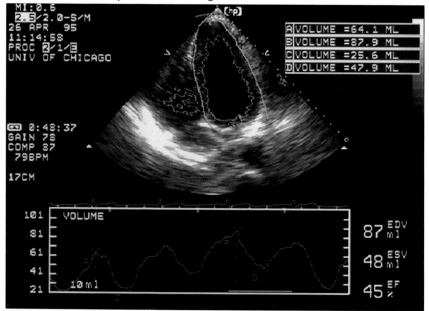

Figure 2.8. Diagram depicting significant respirophasic variation in the AQ waveforms in a patient with shortness of breath. Considering three consecutive beats, the end-diastolic volume increases from 64 to 88 mL, illustrating the importance of recording AQ data during held end-expiration when necessary.

Discrepancies Between AQ and Ventriculography

In some cases, AQ volumes have been noted to underestimate ventriculographic volumes. This underestimation is possibly due to one or a combination of the following explanations: 1) ventriculographic volumes may be slightly greater than AQ volumes because the dye fills in the small cavities of the trabeculae of the ventricular walls, and the papillary muscles and mitral valve apparatus are

J.E. Bednarz et al.

excluded, 2) a foreshortened apical image will underestimate echocardiographic volumes, 3) translational or rotational changes in the plane of imaging may differ when comparing angiographic and echocardiographic data, 4) the technical problem of beam width inaccuracies may in some cases widen an endocardial border resulting in an underestimation of echocardiographic volumes, 5) echocardiographic artifact within the LV chamber may be erroneously interpreted by AQ as tissue, and AQ will consequently underestimate volumes (this artifact may be dependent on transducer position), 6) the AQ gain setting selected by the operator is not always optimal at all times during the cardiac cycle, possibly resulting in a slight overestimation of end-systolic volumes and/or a slight underestimation of end-diastolic volumes. A solution could be the use of an electrocardiogram-triggered, time variable gain setting [12].

With experience and consideration of the aforementioned technical factors influencing AQ study quality, one can obtain optimal AQ data which can provide valuable clinical information for patient management. In addition, these AQ techniques are the foundation for performing high quality Color Kinesis studies to assess the timing and magnitude of regional and global endocardial motion (see Chapters 10 and 11).

References

1. Cao Q, Ramadurai M, Hsu T, Pandian N. Factors influencing realtime automated border detection and acoustic quantification and practical tips for optimal analysis of ventricular function. *J Am Soc Echocardiogr* 1992;5:335 (Abstract).
2. *HP Sonos Phased Array Imaging System User's Guide: System's Basics*, Hewlett-Packard Company, Andover, MA.
3. Perez JE, Waggoner AD, Barzilai B, Melton HE, Miller JG, Sobel BE. On-line assessment of ventricular function by automatic boundary detection and ultrasonic backscatter imaging. *J Am Coll Cardiol* 1992;19:313-20.
4. Vandenberg BF, Rath LS, Stuhlmuller P, Melton HE, Skorton DJ. Estimation of left ventricular cavity area with an on-line, semi-automated echocardiographic edge detection system. *Circulation* 1992;86:159-66.
5. Vandenberg BF, Cardona H, Miller JG, Skorton DJ, Perez JE. On-line left ventricular volume measurement in patients using automated border detection: comparison with conventional echocardiography (multicenter trial) *Circulation* 1992;86:262 (Abstract).

6. Morrissey RL, Siu SC, Guerrero JL, Newell JB, Weyman AE, Picard MH. Automated assessment of ventricular volume and function by echocardiography: validation of automated border detection. *J Am Soc Echocardiogr* 1994;7:107-115.

7. Morrissey RL, Siu SC, Guerrero JL, Weyman AE, Picard MH. Ventricular volume by echocardiographic automated border detection: on-line calculation without loss of accuracy. *J Am Coll Cardiol* 1993;21:275A (Abstract).

8. Gorcsan J III, Deneault LG, Morita S, Kawai A, Griffith BP, Kormos RL. Two-dimensional echocardiographic automated border detection accurately reflects changes in true left ventricular volume. *J Am Coll Cardiol* 1992;19:299A (Abstract).

9. Stewart WJ, Rodkey S, Gunawardena S, White R, Luvisi B, Klein A, Salcedo E. Left ventricular volume calculation with integrated backscatter from echocardiography. *J Am Soc Echocardiogr* 1993;6:553-63.

10. Lindower PD, Rath L, Preslar J, Burns TL, Rezai K, Vandenberg B. Acoustic quantification of left ventricular function: comparison with isotope ventriculography. *J Am Soc Echocardiogr* 1992;5:335 (Abstract).

11. Cao Q, Azevedo J, Snapper H, Schwartz S, Udelson J, Pandian N. Automated, on-line determination of left ventricular volumes and ejection fraction by acoustic quantification: 1) *in vitro* validation, 2) *in vivo* comparison with radionuclide method in patients, 3) examination of factors influencing its accuracy, and 4) clinical application. *J Am Coll Cardiol* 1993;21:275 (Abstract).

12. Marcus RH, Bednarz JE, Coulden R, Shroff S, Lipton M, Lang RM. Ultrasonic backscatter system for automated on-line endocardial boundary detection: evaluation by ultrafast computed tomography. *J Am Coll Cardiol* 1993;22:839-47.

13. Weyman AE. *Principles and Practice of Echocardiography*. 2nd ed. Philadelphia, PA: Lea & Febiger, 1994:106-116.

14. Perez JE, Klein SC, Prater DM, Fraser CE, Cardona H, Waggoner AD, Holland MR, Miller JG, Sobel BE. Automated, on-line quantification of left ventricular dimensions and function by echocardiography with backscatter imaging and lateral gain compensation. *Am J Cardiol* 1992;70:1200-05.

15. Waggoner AD, Miller JG, Perez JE. Two-dimensional echocardiographic automatic boundary detection for evaluation of left ventricular function in unselected adult patients. *J Am Soc Echocardiogr* 1994;7:459-64.

16. Tutt LK, Kopelen HA, Vukovic HA, Soto JG, Zoghbi WA, Quinones MA. Acoustic quantification of fractional area change of the left ventricle: reproducibility of results between technologists in a non-selected cardiac population. *Circulation* 1992;86:262 (Abstract).

3 Comparative and Validation Studies of Echocardiographic On-line Quantification of Left Ventricular Dimensions and Systolic Function

Julio E. Pérez

The impact of echocardiography in clinical practice stems from its inherent ability to provide information regarding cardiac dimensions and, therefore, correlative indices of cardiac structure and function [1]. Thus, M-Mode derived measurements of right and left ventricular thickness, internal dimensions of ventricles and left atrium and ventricular mass gained acceptance by clinicians [2] and have been an essential component of the echocardiography report, as part of the cardiovascular evaluation of patients. The introduction of two-dimensional echocardiography enabled the acquisition of more precise measurements [3], and recent implementation of three dimensional echocardiography [4] promise even more accurate measurements of cavity and wall dimensions and chamber function. Despite this recognized potential and the introduction of image digitization and cine loop capabilities, it has been difficult to implement the routine measurement of ventricular dimensions and function from two dimensional images in day-to-day practice because of time constraints. The American Society of Echocardiography has published a document that provides guidelines for performing these measurements [5] but these have not been widely adopted because off line analysis of images is time-consuming and is typically based on only one representative cardiac cycle. It is common practice to obtain M-Mode derived measurements of left ventricular dimensions and provide a visual assessment of ventricular volumes and ejection fraction. Although visual estimates of ventricular function are reliable when performed by experienced observers, reliable and reproducible quantification based on two dimensional images is essential because of the limitations of M-Mode techniques and inter-observer variability related to the experience of the observer. Computer-assisted detection of the boundary between the blood pool and endocardium has been a long-standing goal of echocardiography. Several investigators have employed digital, computer-generated image reconstruction from the gray level video information, either in single frame or sequentially stored frames with high success [6-13]. Despite their unquestionable merit, these applications that require off-line computer processing have been largely utilized by a single group, or groups of investigators but have not gained acceptance in commercialized products to be widely utilized at present.

In parallel, there has been continued progress in the quantitative characterization of myocardial acoustic properties via the measurement of tissue integrated backscatter [14] that has evolved into a real time imaging technique for clinical investigations. This approach, which is being developed to complement conventional echocardiography, is based on the measurement (in dB) of the power along each radiofrequency line in the field of view before this quantitative information is relayed to the scan converter for the creation of the image. This quantitative image processing approach typically employs an integration time (3.2 μs), longer than that used in conventional echo-cardiography which yields images with considerable reduction in speckle. This property lends itself for facilitating the recognition between blood pool (very low scattering) and endocardium boundary (relatively much higher scattering) in each frame of the image to allow on-line differentiation of blood pool areas in real time [15-17].

Thus, the implementation of this approach has opened a new line of investigations and clinical applications in echocardiography by removing the subjectivity of the visual interpretation of cardiac size and function from the opinions of experts, and incorporating the role of the sonographers in the laboratory acquiring the images [18] in ensuring optimal technical imaging conditions to obtain the measurements at the time of the examination. In addition, a real-time physiological display of the resultant cavity area dimensions and functional indexes has been introduced for the first time in echocardiography. Although originally employed, the term "automatic" boundary detection (ABD) may not truly describe the manner in which the system operates as the sonographer's role continues to be essential for selection of the cardiac chambers of interest for study and for optimizing image quality (commercial name is Acoustic Quantification® or, briefly, AQ). Nevertheless, these on-line measurements of cardiovascular function have received considerable attention in the last 5 years since the introduction of the first commercial product and the purpose of this chapter is to review these applications and the comparative studies against independent correlative techniques that have validated the use of on-line quantification of cardiac function by echocardiography.

Ventricular Size and Function On-line

Validation by Off-line Analysis of Conventional Two-Dimensional Transthoracic Echocardiography

Initial work in our laboratory focused on measurement of left ventricular cavity areas at end diastole and end systole from short axis and apical four chamber views and the measurement of left ventricular fractional area change [19] by transthoracic imaging. We studied 54 patients and 12 normal subjects with broad ranges of ventricular dimensions and systolic function. The cavity areas and the fractional area change measured on-line correlated well with the areas and ejection fraction measured off line, respectively. More than 70% of patients and subjects could be studied adequately. In this study we realized the importance of calculating the cavity areas off-line by manual tracing in the very same cardiac cycle (simultaneous beats) that yielded the measurements on-line in order to obtain a fair comparison (Figure 3.1). In the practice of echo-cardiography the observer who provides the interpretation tends to ignore the effects of respiration and patient motion-induced image artifacts to produce a "time-average" visual assessment of cavity size and function. We learned that on-line quantification is obviously "sensitive" to these influences. This is not surprising as the same effects occur in all modalities of echocardiography (such as is the case of Doppler echocardiography, i.e. changes in peak flow velocity) when the exact position of the transducer with respect to the region of interest is not maintained over the cardiac cycle.

J.E. Pérez

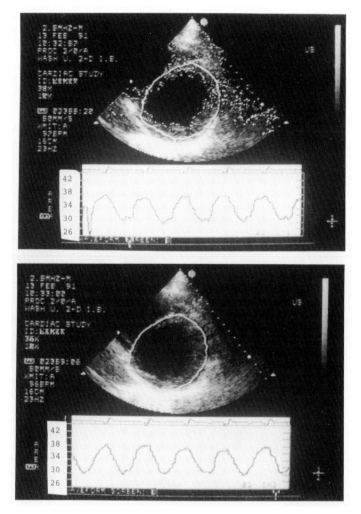

Figure 3.1. Top: Short axis boundary detected image with the on-line instantaneous LV cavity area signal calculated within a circular region of interest drawn through the mid-myocardium (bright line). Bottom: Images obtained with the AQ software running in the background without displaying the detected boundary, were recorded on tape for off-line analysis. The analysis included manual tracing of the endocardial boundary and the calculation of the cross-sectional area of the LV cavity. Results were compared with those of the automated detection obtained from the simultaneously recorded LV area signals. (Reproduced with permission from the American College of Cardiology, Pérez JE *et al.*, *J Am Coll Cardiol* 1992;19:313-320)

In additional studies, Vandenberg *et al.*. [20] compared the new on-line method with off-line manually traced cavity areas (non simultaneous beats) in 8 normal subjects. Specifically, under conditions of higher transmit gain there was a good correlation among manually traced and on-line cavity areas (r=0.92; Figure 3.2) but the manually drawn areas were underestimated by the on-line system. Under conditions of low-gain settings the manually drawn areas were overestimated by the on-line method and the correlation was lower (r=0.79) whereas with intermediate gain settings there was an acceptable correlation (r=0.91). Thus, these investigators determined that the method was reproducible although (as stated above) like all of the echocardiography modalities, it was gain-dependent. A collaborative study between The University of Iowa and Washington University [21] reported on the first implementation of left ventricular derived on-line mediated by the conversion of cavity areas into volumes by either the modified Simpson's method, area-length determination (utilizing both apical views) and the ellipsoid approximation (short axis views) in 42 patients. The correlations were made against off-line derived volumes by tracing the endocardial borders in a workstation. The correlations were excellent (r=0.97, r=0.99, and r=0.91 for end-diastolic, end-systolic and ejection fraction, respectively) albeit only 43% of patients met the selection criterion of having better than 75% endocardial border tracking to make the images suitable for off-line tracing and on-line determination of volumes.

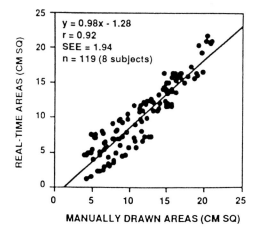

Figure 3.2. Scatterplot shows comparison of real-time and manually drawn areas in the high-gain training group (non-simultaneous beats, all subjects, including those with high cavity clutter). (Reproduced with permission from the American Heart Association, Vandenberg *et al.*, *Circulation* 1992;86:159-166).

Additional work in this related topic was carried out by Mugge and coworkers [22] who compared on-line measurements of cavity areas with off-line tracings of the endocardial boundaries in 42 patients and found excellent correlations (r=0.78, 0.84 and 0.84 for end-diastolic, end-systolic areas and fractional area change, respectively, in apical views) and similar results in short axis views. In other studies by Herregods and collaborators [23] the on-line method was compared with off-line measurements in conventional echo-cardiographic images (non-simultaneous). For the group of 75 patients and normal subjects the left ventricular end-diastolic area was significantly smaller by the on-line method as compared to the off-line manual tracing approach (both for the short axis and apical views). The end-systolic areas were larger, and the resulting fractional area change was smaller than that obtained with the off-line manual tracing technique (Figure 3.3). The authors attributed the differences to the strong influence of gain adjustments needed in the system utilized at that time (no lateral gain compensation was available at that time and studies were not controlled from changes in transducer position and location in the chest wall). In addition, the detection of the components of the mitral valve apparatus within the ventricular cavity subtracts from the true diastolic volume and further contributes to the underestimation in that phase of the cardiac cycle.

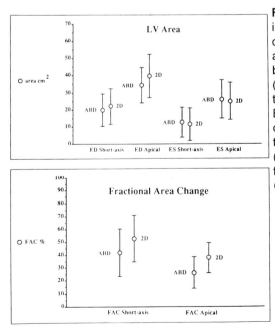

Figure 3.3. Analysis of data in 75 patients and subjects; comparisons of on-line LV area measurement with the boundary detection method (ABD) vs. off-line manual tracing (ED - end-diastole, ES - end-systole, 2D - two-dimensional, FAC - frac-tional area change). (Reproduced with permission from Herregods *et al.*, *Am J Cardiol* 1993;72:359-362).

In summary, the above mentioned studies employed primarily conventional echocardiography with off-line manual tracing of endocardial boundaries to validate the on-line system. Other studies, mentioned below, that pursued other types of validation, also utilized this type of comparative analysis, but to a lesser extent.

Validation by Off-line Analysis of Conventional Transesophageal Echocardiography

In two separate studies Cao and coworkers [24,25] determined the value of employing lateral gain compensation (a new approach designed to optimize image quality developed for this application; Figure 3.4) for improved detection and on-line tracking of the endocardial boundaries by both transthoracic (25 patients) and transesophageal multiplane echocardiography (20 patients). Torrecilla and collaborators [26] also documented good correlations between on-line and off-line measurements for left ventricular cavity areas and fractional area change during either transthoracic and transesophageal imaging, although, as expected, the correlations were superior for the latter imaging modality with better delineation of the endocardial-blood boundary. In other studies, Stoddard *et al.* [27] studied 38 consecutive patients with on-line determination of left ventricular cavity areas by transesophageal echocardiography. They demonstrated the feasibility to obtain accurate images in 92% of 95% of patients from the short axis and four-chamber views, respectively. They obtained excellent correlations between on-line cavity areas and off-line traced areas. The use of lateral gain compensation significantly improved the comparisons between left ventricular cavity area measurements obtained on-line and those obtained by manual tracing of transesophageal echocardiography images using a biplane probe. In similar studies Dávila-Román *et al.* [28] obtained transesophageal images in 16 patients from the short axis view and in 9 patients studied from a longitudinal plane with excellent correlations (r=0.9) achieved for all comparisons.

Thus, the use of on-line quantification of cavity size and function appeared to perform even better when employing transesophageal imaging with the improvement in image quality that this modality confers. This was extended to applications that included intraoperative monitoring as will be discussed later in this chapter.

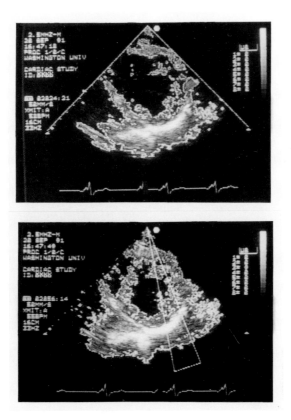

Figure 3.4. Top: short axis view of the left ventricle at the level of the papillary muscle with border detection delineating the lateral borders only poorly (arrows) because of anisotropic properties of myocardium. Bottom: same image but with the lateral gain compensation enhancement sector located over the first region of myocardium to be enhanced selectively. Facing page, top: after selective lateral gain compensation of the posteroseptal wall the endocardium is readily

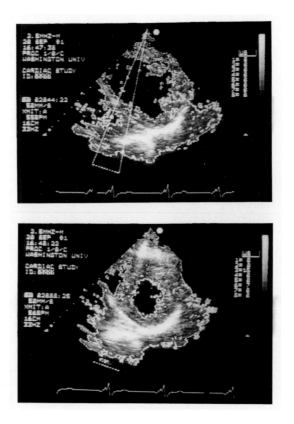

detected and tracked, even though the anterolateral wall remains delineated only poorly. Bottom: after selective enhancement of the anterolateral wall (with a procedure similar to that described above), the endocardium is now well detected and the image is now suitable for on-line quantification. (Reproduced with permission from Pérez *et al.*, *Am J Cardiol* 1992;70:1200-1205).

Validation By Radionuclide Ventriculography

Because of the general success of radionuclide ventriculography in obtaining measurement of left ventricular ejection fraction in all patients it is not surprising that it has been utilized by several investigators to compare the measurements derived by on-line echocardiography. Lindower and coworkers [29] initially reported in preliminary studies the evaluation of 19 patients by both radionuclide ventriculography and on-line determination of left ventricular cavity areas and fractional area change by echocardiography (Figure 3.5).

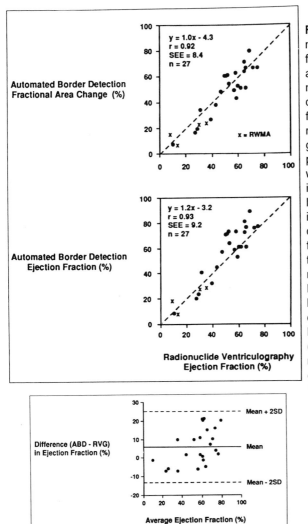

Figure 3.5. Top and middle: Plots of fractional area change and ejection fraction as measured by border detection vs. ejection fraction measured by radio-nuclide ventriculography (RVG); x= patients with regional wall motion abnormalities (RWMA). Dashed line is the line of identity. Bottom: Limits of agreement of ejection fraction determined by the border detection method (ABD) and RVG. Ejection fraction by ABD tended to overestimate that by RVG as it increased. (Reproduced with permission from Lindower et al., *Am J Cardiol* 1994;73:195-199).

In 74% of patients there was adequate image quality to obtain the measurements by echocardiography and the correlation with radionuclide technique was highly significant (r=0.93, p<0.0001). San Román *et al.* [30] also documented a good correlation between ejection fraction measured by radionuclide ventriculography and fractional area change measured by on-line echocardiography (r=0.89, p=0.0013) in 10 patients. In another study, 20 patients underwent simultaneous radionuclide ventriculography and on-line echocardiographic volume determination [31] and good correlations were obtained (r=0.8 for end-diastolic volumes, r=0.90 for end-systolic volumes and r=0.92 for ejection fraction). Further validation of the measurement of fractional area change obtained directly by the on-line measurement system was derived from studies by Gorcsan *et al.* [32] who studied 88 consecutive patients aged 53±14 years undergoing radionuclide ventriculography for measurement of ejection fraction (Figure 3.6). Short axis echocardiographic views were obtained to measure end-diastolic and end-systolic cavity areas and fractional area change. In addition, the left ventricular major axis was measured from apical views and was used to derive echocardiographic volumes and ejection fraction by the area-length and the Simpson's method. Technically adequate images were obtained in 78% of patients and correlations with radionuclide techniques were acceptable (r=0.84 for fractional area change vs. ejection fraction, r=0.89 for area-length ejection fraction vs. radionuclide ejection fraction and r=0.91 for Simpson's vs. radionuclide ejection fraction).

Further comparisons with radionuclide ventriculography were provided in completed studies by Lindower *et al.* [33] in 27 of 46 patients in whom adequate image quality was obtained (>75% endocardial detection and tracking during real time imaging). Fractional area change measured from the short axis views correlated well with ejection fraction by radionuclide ventriculography (r=0.92, standard error of the estimate of 8.4%). The ejection fraction derived from the short axis echocardiographic data by a modified ellipsoid model showed a strong linear correlation with that determined by the radionuclide method (r=0.90, standard error of 9.5%; see Figure 3.6) in 23 of the patients without severe wall motion abnormalities.

Further comparisons of the accuracy to measure the ejection fraction as compared to radionuclide ventriculography were reported in studies published by Yvorchuk *et al.* [34]. In 54 patients they compared the measurement of left ventricular ejection fraction by the on-line echocardiographic method vs. that determined by radionuclide ventriculography (non-simultaneous). There were good correlations for both the data obtained from the apical four-chamber view (r=0.89, n=43) and apical two-chamber view (r=0.83, n=26). There was a better correlation as more experience was acquired in obtaining the echocardiography images (last 30 patients studied, r=0.91, n=25 four-chamber views, and r=0.86, n=16 for the apical two-chamber views). Although the correlations were good, there was a tendency of the echocardiographic method to underestimate the values obtained by radionuclide ventriculography (mean difference among the two techniques of less than zero).

Thus, the assessment of either fractional area change or ejection fraction by on-line quantification by echocardiography is reasonably accurate when compared with results obtained by radionuclide ventriculography despite of the fact that the data is acquired in a non-simultaneous manner and the disparity among the two approaches (i.e. counts vs. area-based determination).

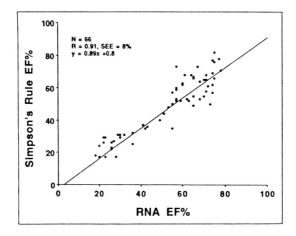

Figure 3.6. Relation of Simpson's rule ejection fraction (EF) using the border detection method from short axis data to radionuclide (RNA) left ventricular ejection fraction. (Reproduced with permission from Gorcsan *et al.*, *Am J Cardiol* 1993;72:810-815).

Validation by Contrast Cineventriculography

Comparisons with data obtained by cineventriculography were provided by Epperlein *et al.* [35] who studied 15 unselected patients who were undergoing cardiac catheterization. The left ventricular end-diastolic volumes by the on-line technique correlated well with the off-line tracing of the two-dimensional images (mean of 107.1±39.5 ml vs. 114.4±41.3, r=0.93) although were underestimated with respect to catheterization (180.4±35.2 ml, r=0.87 with the on-line method although with a standard error of the estimate of 23.5 ml). The end-systolic volumes were smaller by the on-line technique as compared to catheterization (56.7±35.2 vs. 84.7±64.3 ml, r=0.89). The ejection fraction averaged 49.8±10.4% by the on-line method and 58.5±12.8 % by catheterization (r=0.76, standard error of the estimate of 11.3%). There was no further analysis provided in this study regarding the relative bias between values obtained by the two methods which would have provided additional insight in the comparative analysis. Studies by Vanoverschelde *et al.* [36] compared left ventricular volumes and ejection fraction in 36 patients measured by the on-line echocardiography method and by cineventriculography (Figure 3.7). The on-line echocardiography method underestimated the end-diastolic volumes (131±57 vs. 159±64 ml by ventriculography, r=0.78) although the correlation was better for end-systolic volumes (r=0.9, albeit with a large standard error of the estimate of 20.4 ml). The ejection fraction showed a correlation coefficient of r=0.87 with a standard error of only 5% (mean values of 35±11 vs. 39±13%). The underestimation of left ventricular volumes by any modality that utilizes echocardiography as compared to cineventriculography is well known and is attributable to various inherent differences in the techniques (see Chapter 2). Among these one can enumerate: the use of contrast opacification of the chamber versus the outlining of the endocardium silhouette in two dimension, underestimation of the true major axis (foreshortening in the apical views), difficulties with visualization of any apical segments (whether the image is foreshortened or not), the use of single plane echocardiography approximation as opposed to a more precise but less practical biplanar approach and the inclusion of the papillary muscles and mitral valve tissue in the echocardiographic images that tend to subtract from the volumes otherwise estimated by contrast ventriculography. Therefore, it is not surprising to obtain underestimation of the ventricular volumes by the on-line echocardiographic method against those derived by contrast ventriculography. Nevertheless, the close estimates obtained for the measurement of ejection fraction as shown [36] validates this application with the new echocardiographic method.

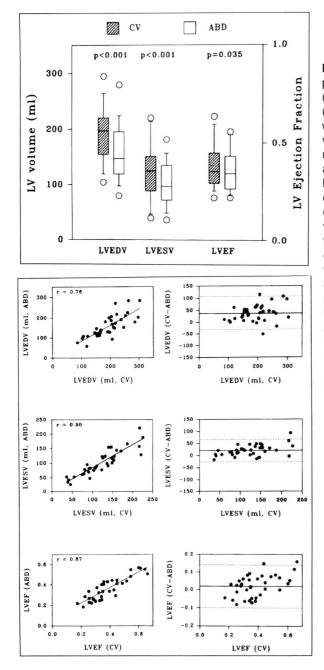

Figure 3.7. Top: Box plots showing mean (dotted lines) ± 1 SD (box range), along with the median values (solid lines), range (open circles) and 95% confidence limits for LV end-diastolic (ED) and end-systolic (ES) volumes and ejection fraction (EF) by contrast cine-ventriculography (CV) and ABD. Bottom, left, scatterplots showing the relation between ABD and CV left ventricular ED volume (top), ES volume (center), and ejection fraction (bottom). Bottom, right: residual plot analysis showing the distribution of the residuals (CV-ABD) as a function of· CV volumes measured at end-diastole (top), end-systole (center), and CV ejection fraction (bottom). (Reproduced with permission from Vanoverschelde *et al.*, *Am J Cardiol* 1994;74:633-635).

Validation by Ultrafast Computed Tomography

Further clarification of the need for refinements in the original design of the on-line echocardiography measurement system were provided by studies authored by Marcus *et al.* [37] who studied 10 subjects with this method and subsequently with ultrafast computed tomography (non-simultaneous). Measurements of left ventricular cavity area were compared at end-diastole and end-systole and time course analyses of cavity area during the cardiac cycle. There was good correlation between values for end-diastolic area (r=0.99) end-systolic area (r=0.91) and fractional area change (r=0.91) using the two methods. The on-line system underestimated the end-diastolic area (small negative bias of -1.6 cm²) but with narrow confidence limits (-3.6 cm² to 0.4 cm²). The end-systolic area was overestimated by the echocardiography measurement (small positive bias of 2.6 cm²) but with wider confidence intervals (7.9 to -2.8 cm²). Real time values for fractional area change were 13% smaller than those determined by ultrafast computed tomography. The authors attributed the observed differences to alterations in gain sensitivity of the system over the cardiac cycle (Figure 3.8) and suggested that an electrocardiographic-triggered time-varying gain control may further improve accuracy of the measurements.

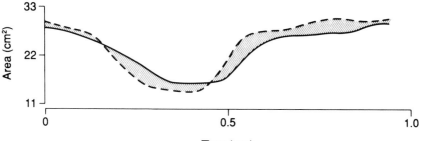

Figure 3.8. Area-time plots obtained using ultrafast computed tomography (dashed curve) and acoustic quantification (on-line measurement by echocardiography-solid curve) in a representative subject. The duration of systole measured from the peak of the R wave of the ECG to end-systole (minimal cavity area) was longer for the real time data (436±53 ms) than for ultrafast computed tomographic measurements (372±39 ms, p<0.01). This effect contributed to the observed differences among the two measurements. (Reproduced with permission from Marcus *et al.*, *J Am Coll Cardiol* 1993;22:839-847).

Validation By Magnetic Resonance Imaging

Studies by Stewart *et al.* [38] provided further validation for the new methodology. They studied 27 patients by on-line echocardiographic quantification, of which 12 underwent magnetic resonance imaging of the heart to determine the left ventricular volumes as well. The investigators employed an approach based on a modification of the Pappus' theorem which states that the volume of a solid object formed by rotating a cross-sectional area around a central axis (not intersecting the area) is the product of that area times the distance traveled by the centroid of that region. This approximation permitted calculation of the ventricular volume by summing the individual components that were modeled as wedge-shaped slices (in this case 12 slices). In addition, the authors derived ventricular volumes by an approximation of the summated ellipsoid method, by hand-drawn borders from the images. The measurements obtained with on-line echocardiography correlated well with those using a standard biplane area-length method derived off-line from endocardial borders drawn by hand from the same echocardiographic data (r=0.95). Furthermore, volumes derived from the on-line method from six imaging planes with both the Pappus' rule and the summated ellipsoid method correlated well with the volumes derived from magnetic resonance imaging (r=0.91 and r=0.90, respectively), whereas the use of one imaging plane correlated less well (r=0.75). Thus, the method was extensively validated (Figure 3.9) but this study again emphasized the importance of employing at least a biapical (or multiple plane) imaging to obtain the most accurate information about ventricular volumes and, therefore, the derived indices of function with the on-line method.

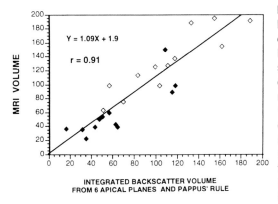

INTEGRATED BACKSCATTER VOLUME
FROM 6 APICAL PLANES AND PAPPUS' RULE

Figure 3.9. Comparison of LV volume measurements obtained with AQ and the Pappus' rule method from six apical views with those obtained with magnetic resonance imaging (MRI) in 12 patients. End-diastole - open diamonds; end-systole - closed diamonds. (Reprinted with permission from Stewart *et al., J Am Soc Echocardiogr* 1993; 6:553-563).

Validation With Measurements By Electromagnetic Flow Meter

In order to validate the accuracy of the on-line quantitative echocardiographic approach Gorcsan *et al.* [39] compared the changes in left ventricular cavity area from end-diastole to end-systole (echo stroke area) measured from open-chest dogs against the directly measured left ventricular stroke volume measured by an electromagnetic flow probe placed in the ascending aorta. The stroke volume was recorded from the same cardiac cycle in which the echocardiographic area change was measured during episodes of apnea in the experimental animal and during occlusions of the inferior vena cava. Changes in echocardiographic stroke area correlated closely with changes in left ventricular stroke volume for 540 matched beats (r=0.93, SEE=5%). Thus, alterations in stroke volume could be closely approximated by the on-line echocardiographic measurement system in this experimental animal preparation.

Determinations of True Volumes in Isolated Heart Preparations, Explanted Hearts or by Means of Three-Dimensional Echocardiography

Studies by Morrissey *et al.* [40] employed a beating canine heart model in which an intracavitary balloon was placed to continuously control and measure the actual volume of the cavity. The on-line echocardiographic measurements of ventricular volumes were compared against the off-line manually traced images, and the actual volumes from the direct measurement (altered within a range of 7-92 ml). There was an excellent correlation between the on-line and off-line methods (r=0.91) and both methods equally underestimated the actual volumes because of the difficulty in obtaining the true longitudinal plane. Results of this study are applicable to the practice of echocardiography where the true major axis of the left ventricle is frequently not obtained in patients when imaging from apical views.

Studies by Cao *et al.* [31] provided important validation studies for on-line determined left ventricular volumes and systolic function. First, 25 symmetric and asymmetric-shaped canine hearts were imaged in a water bath and volumes were derived by the border detection method. Then, absolute ventricular volumes were measured by volume displacement with saline obtaining excellent correlations among the methods (r=0.99).

With respect to left ventricular aneurysms, Azevedo *et al.* [41] employed the on-line echocardiographic system to determine the area of the aneurysms and volume was compared *in vitro* (excised hearts of dogs with ventricular aneurysms). Also these investigators studied 20 patients with apical aneurysms measured by on-line echocardiography and compared the results with those derived from three-dimensional echocardiographic reconstructions. The on-line measurement of the aneurysm area compared well with the direct measurements or the three-dimensional reconstructions.

Additional information regarding underestimation of volumes by the on-line border detection method was obtained from comparisons made by Jiang and coworkers [42] who compared the ventricular volumes obtained by the on-line method (presumably single plane images) with three-dimensional reconstructions made in 13 animal hearts. Although good correlations were obtained (r=0.88) underestimation was significant (39±10%).

After their preliminary results [40] more definitive studies by Morrissey *et al.* [43] again highlighted the importance of optimal image quality, not different from any other echocardiography modality, when performing on-line quantification of left ventricular volumes and ejection fraction. They employed an experimental canine heart preparation with extracorporeal pumping an oxygenation, where a latex balloon was positioned inside the left ventricle and known aliquots of colored water were added as measured from a fluid column. Thus, it was possible to know exactly the intraventricular (intra-balloon) volume at all times (including alterations over a wide range) in this beating heart preparation. Measurements obtained by the on-line system were compared to off-line manual tracings of the cavity and to the true volumes measured directly in the animal preparation as described above. Over a wide range of volumes (12-127 ml) the measurements obtained on-line were correlated (r=0.81) to the true volumes, but with a high standard error of the estimate (13.5 ml), whereas the off-line method correlated better with true volumes (r=0.96, standard error of 6.7 ml). Nevertheless, the correlation for ejection fraction was much better (r=0.94, standard error of 4.3%) which was not different from that obtained by off-line tracings (Figure 3.10). The authors concluded that, despite the variability observed in volumes, the close correlation for ejection fraction and the rapid features of the system make it potentially very useful in the clinical setting.

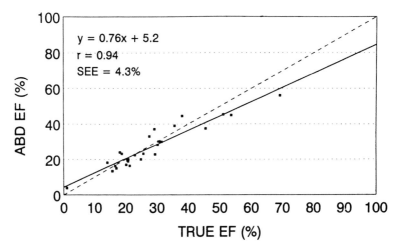

Figure 3.10. Correlation of ejection fraction (EF) by on-line ABD (border detection method) and true ejection fraction. SEE - standard error of the estimate; dashed line - line of identity; solid line - regression line. (Reproduced with permission from Morrissey *et al.*, *J Am Soc Echocardiogr* 1994;7:105-115.)

Validation of Dimensions with the Use of Implanted Sonomicrometers

Paulsen and coworkers [44] compared on-line echocardiographic measurements of left ventricular cavity area against direct measurements by implanted ultrasonic crystals in dogs obtaining good correlations. They also measured the rate of left ventricular cavity emptying and filling at baseline and in response to dobutamine and esmolol, sequentially. The correlation for indices of emptying (r=0.8) was better than for the indices of ventricular filling (r=0.67).

Feasibility Studies in Consecutive Patients and Assessment of Reproducibility of Results

As mentioned and illustrated before (Figure 3.4), lateral gain compensation was developed in order to minimize the dependence of the echocardiography system's gain over the quality of the images [45]. In order to evaluate the feasibility of performing these measurements and their reproducibility in the same subject, we obtained on-line echocardiographic quantitative images in 60 control subjects and 10 patients with cardiac dysfunction. The use of lateral gain compensation, allowed optimization of the system's gain in the lateral and medial aspects of the image (i.e. lateral wall and apical septum in apical views) without compromising the low gain which is appropriate for the blood pool cavity. With this approach, we determined the range for normal values of left ventricular cavity area and function in the short axis views (13.1±3.7 cm² and 5.9±2.7 cm² at end-diastole and end-systole, respectively, with fractional area change of 55.6±11.2%) and apical four chamber views (23.8±4.5 cm² and 15.5±3.4 cm² at end-diastole and end-systole, respectively, with fractional area change of 34.7±7.8%). The peak instantaneous rate of cavity area change averaged 50 cm²/s in systole and 60 cm²/s in diastole, in each view in normal subjects. Serial measurements carried out in the same subjects (individuals who were not taking medications that would alter loading conditions in any significant way) over a 3 week interval yielded highly reproducible results (Figure 3.11).

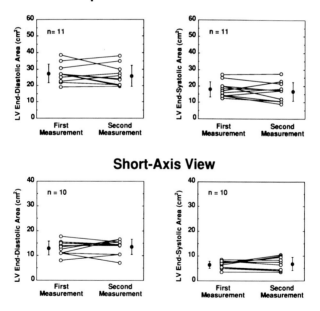

Figure 3.11. Reproducibility of sequential LV cavity area determinations on-line in 2 separate studies in apical and short axis views at end-diastole (left panels) and end-systole (right panels) at intervals of 2 to 3 weeks in each subject. Mean values ± SD on the two studies were virtually identical. (Reproduced with permission from Pérez *et al.*, *Am J Cardiol* 1992;70:1200-1205).

When we studied patients with dilated cardiomyopathy they exhibited values for cavity area averaging 49.1±6.1 cm² and 43.1±4.9 cm² for end-diastole and end-systole, respectively, with fractional area change averaging 12.2±3.0% in the apical views. Thus, on-line echocardiographic backscatter imaging-assisted endocardial boundary detection was possible, reproducible and offered quantitative indices of function at the bedside.

Improved reproducibility in measurements of left ventricular cavity areas as obtained by various sonographers was reported by Tutt *et al.* [46] as long as transthoracic imaging provided good quality recordings with adequate endocardial detection and tracking over the cardiac cycle.

In studies published by Waggoner *et al.* [47] 68 consecutive patients were studied by the on-line echocardiography method to assess its feasibility in unselected patients and to compare its ability to detect and track specific endocardial segments. From each view (short axis, apical four-chamber and apical two-chamber views) the left ventricle was divided in 6 endocardial segments. The short axis view was successfully obtained in 53 of the 68 patients; of the possible 318 segments, 96% were visualized by conventional echocardiography and 89% by the border detection method. From the apical four-chamber view (obtained in 63 of the 68 patients) conventional echocardiography visualized 93% of segments vs. 86% by the border detection method. In the apical two-chamber view (obtained in 58 of the 68 patients) the respective values for successfully obtaining the images were 88% and 80%, respectively. Overall, the border detection technique detected all six segments in 73, 72 and 72% of the short axis, four chamber and two chamber views, respectively. Discrepancies between the two techniques (detected by two dimensional but not able to be tracked well by the border detection technique) were found in the short axis inferior and lateral wall segments, four-chamber lateral wall and two-chamber anterior wall (Figure 3.12). In the study group there were 46 patients with normal wall motion and 33 patients with segmental wall motion abnormalities. The time required (in addition to the time spent obtaining conventional images as part of a routine study) to perform an examination of endocardial border detection averaged 375 seconds (range 180 to 780 sec). Thus, the utilization of the endocardial border detection technique was associated with a clinically acceptable frequency of visualization of left ventricular segments given that adequate (not necessarily excellent) conventional image quality is obtained.

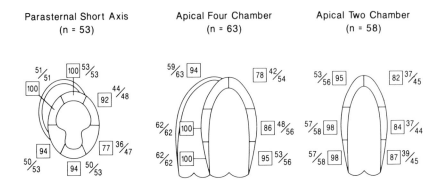

Figure 3.12. Success of ABD (border detection, on-line method) segmental left ventricular imaging expressed on the basis of suitable visualization first by conventional echocardiographic imaging. Values of n represents number of consecutive patients studied by each imaging plane from transthoracic windows. Numbers inside the boxes are percent of patients in whom there was first adequate visualization by conventional imaging and then detection of segment by ABD imaging as well (fraction yields percent). (Reproduced with permission from Waggoner *et al.*, *J Am Soc Echocardiogr* 1994;7:459-464).

Comparison with Correlative M-Mode Derived Cardiac Dimensions and Functional Indexes

As part of a study designed to evaluate the influence that variability in heart rate and respiration exert upon the left ventricular volumes measured on-line, Seliem *et al.* [48] compared the ventricular volumes and ejection fraction derived by the on-line echocardiographic method against the corresponding M-Mode dimensions and fractional shortening in 43 children. Despite the non-simultaneous and indirect comparison (M-mode vs. two-dimensional data) there was a good correlation between end-diastolic dimension by M-Mode (cm) and end-diastolic volume (ml) by the on-line method (r=0.87). Similarly, the end-systolic dimension and the end-systolic volume exhibited a good correlation (r=0.83) as was the case for the fractional shortening (M-Mode) and the ejection fraction (r=0.76).

*Validation by Thermodilution Measurements of Cardiac Output
in Intensive Care Settings*

In preliminary studies [49] Pinto and coworkers validated the on-line
measurements of left ventricular short axis cavity area to derive ventricular
volumes versus cardiac output obtained by transesophageal echocardiography
(combined two-dimensional and Doppler methods) against thermodilution-
determined cardiac output in 8 patients undergoing cardiac surgery.   The
average difference between the two techniques was -0.2±1.3 l/min. and a
correlation coefficient of 0.71 was obtained.   Additional studies by Tardif *et al.*
[50] validated the use on-line determination of cardiac output by the Doppler-
two dimensional echocardiography approach and by thermodilution in critically
ill patients (Figure 3.13).

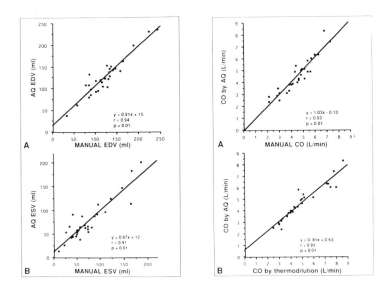

Figure 3. 13. Left: (A) correlation between acoustic quantification and manual
analysis for (A) end-diastolic volume (EDV); and (B) end-systolic volume (ESV).
Right: (A) correlation between acoustic quantification and manual analysis for
cardiac output (CO); and (B) correlation between acoustic quantification and
thermodilution for cardiac output.   (Reproduced with permission from Tardif *et
al., Am J Cardiol* 1994;74:810-813).

In 78% of patients of Tardif's study, images of adequate quality were obtained and there was an excellent correlation between the on-line determination of ventricular volumes and those determined off-line by manual tracing of the images (r=0.94 and 0.91 for end-diastole and end-systole, respectively. The correlation for ejection fraction was 0.85 and for cardiac output by the combined echocardiography-Doppler technique was 0.97. The correlation between on-line echocardiographic measurement of cardiac output and that determined by thermodilution was very good (r=0.95) but the agreement had wide limits (-0.3±1.1 l/min.). A similar underestimation was noted between the Doppler approach and the thermodilution technique leading the authors to conclude that the bias was introduced by the conventional echocardiographic determination and not by the new on-line boundary detection method.

Feinberg *et al.* [51] reported on the use of the border detection technique employed with transesophageal echocardiography in a patient with cardiogenic shock after mitral valve replacement that was managed with a left ventricular assist device. Serial evaluation of left ventricular function was performed with the method for 6 days showing gradual and significant improvement in systolic performance over time as determined from increases in fractional area change (7% at day 2, increasing to 38% at day 6) and who was then able to be weaned from the device at that time. These results suggested a promising role for this method in the bedside determination of the timing for successful removal of mechanical assist devices after surgical interventions.

Studies reported by Sun *et al.* [52] validated the measurement by transthoracic echocardiography of ventricular volumes, ejection fraction and cardiac output in 50 patients in the intensive care unit setting. The left ventricular volumes (end-diastolic, end-systolic) and ejection fraction were calculated by the on-line measurement system and compared with off-line tracing of the images (non-simultaneous beats) and the derived cardiac output (from the product of the stroke volume obtained on-line and heart rate) was compared to that obtained by thermodilution. The on-line measurements exhibited excellent correlation with the off-line hand-drawn approach (end-diastolic volume, r=0.98; end-systolic volume, r=0.98 and ejection fraction, r=0.91). Cardiac output derived by the on-line stroke volume was correlated with the one determined from the two-dimensional images off-line (r=0.84), with that obtained by thermodilution (r=0.83) and with those determined from the Doppler techniques (r=0.75 for aortic valve and r=0.60 for the pulmonic valve). Thus, the measurement system performed adequately when compared with more laborious echocardiographic approaches in this clinical setting, notwithstanding the use of transthoracic imaging and the comparison with non-simultaneous beats (Figure 3.14).

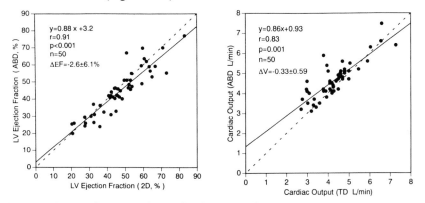

Figure 3.14. Left: comparison of LV ejection fraction by automated boundary detection (ABD) versus two-dimensional echocardiographic methods by linear regression analysis. Right: comparison of cardiac output by ABD and thermodilution (TD) methods by linear regression analysis. (Reproduced with permission from Sun *et al.*, *J Am Soc Echocardiogr* 1995;8:29-36).

Evaluation of the LV Response to Pharmacological Interventions

In other experimental animal preparation Dávila-Roman and coworkers [53] employed the on-line echocardiographic measurement system to assess the myocardial contractile state in dogs with chronic mitral regurgitation by means of the instantaneous peak-systolic pressure/end-systolic area relationship. The slope of the ventricular pressure-area relationship was determined under baseline conditions and after methoxamine or nitroglycerin infusion, and then repeated under conditions of dobutamine stimulation. The slope of the ventricular pressure/area relationship was altered significantly (p=0.0002) and in the expected direction (steeper slope) from baseline to enhanced contractile state after dobutamine infusion. Thus, on-line echocardiographic measurements of ventricular area facilitated the implementation of elastance determinations to serially evaluate the myocardial contractile state under conditions of alterations in preload, afterload and inotropic state. The topic of myocardial contractile state determined by the implementation of measurements of pressure-dimensions relationship via on-line echocardiography is being discussed in more detail in Chapter 9.

Iliceto and coworkers [54] employed the on-line quantification method to evaluate sequential changes in left ventricular cavity area (images obtained from the transthoracic approach) induced by esophageal atrial pacing in 10 patients detecting the physiological reduction in cavity area primarily at end-diastole and to a less extent at end-systole during rapid pacing with return to baseline immediately post-pacing. Next, we studied 27 patients undergoing dobutamine stress echocardiography [55] and successfully obtained images in all patients throughout the infusion of the agent. We observed different responses among patients who had normal wall motion at rest, and who exhibited a visual normal response to dobutamine infusion (hyperdynamic function without wall motion abnormalities), and those who had baseline wall motion abnormalities and either failed to exhibit improved function or developed ischemic responses. In the normal group, end-diastolic cavity areas were reduced modestly at peak dobutamine infusion (by 15%) with marked reductions in end-systolic areas (by 33%), resulting in marked increases in fractional area change (52%) compared to baseline (Figure 3.15). Patients with asynergy (baseline or induced by the agent) had non-significant changes in cavity areas from baseline to peak at both end-diastole and end-systole resulting in blunted response of the fractional area change. The on-line assessment of global LV function during pharmacological stress testing does not minimize the importance of assessment of regional responses, but provides an objective complementary tool for the surveillance of global responses to inotropic stimulation.

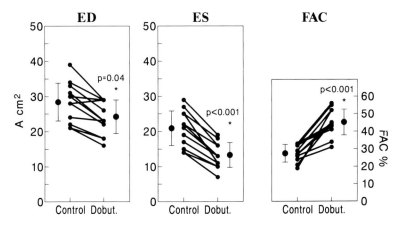

Figure 3.15 (A). Grouped data for patients (n=13) exhibiting a normal response to dobutamine (>30% increment in fractional area change from baseline). A - area; ED - end-diastolic; ES - end-systolic; FAC - fractional area change.

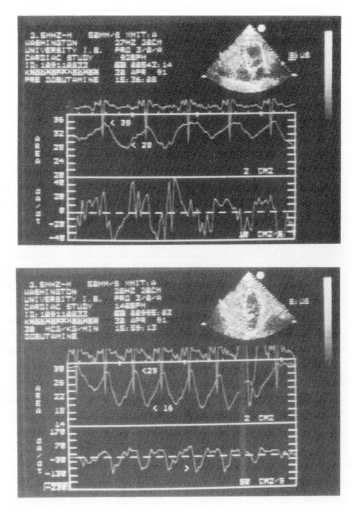

Figure 3.15 (B and C). Baseline and peak dobutamine level area and dA/dt in a patient with normal response to dobutamine infusion. At baseline (top) the peak rate of systolic cavity contraction was at least 40 cm²/s (read as -40 in the left scale of the lower graph of the top image. The baseline diastolic peak rate of expansion averaged 30 cm²/s. After dobutamine (30 µg/kg/min level, bottom) the diastolic and systolic cavity areas are smaller with a marked increase in systolic dA/dt (105 cm²/s; arrowhead; compressed display with calibration now of 50 cm²/s per horizontal division below the dotted zero line) with a peak diastolic rate of expansion of 65 cm²/s. (Reproduced with permission from Pérez *et al., Eur Heart J* 1992;13:1669-1676).

Dubourg and coworkers [56] measured the ability of the on-line measurement system to detect sequential changes in left ventricular dimensions and function in response to nitroglycerin in 13 normal subjects comparing indices of systolic vs. diastolic function.

Validation by a Thermodilution Catheter to Measure Ejection Fraction, and by Intracardiac and Epicardial Echocardiographic Imaging

Excellent correlations were obtained in studies comparing end-diastolic, end-systolic cavity left ventricular cavity areas and fractional area change determined by either intracardiac imaging (5 MHz probe in the right atrium) and epicardial echocardiography in experimental pigs [57]. Schneider and coworkers [58] also demonstrated the feasibility of employing on-line echocardiography measurement of right ventricular cavity areas and fractional area change as compared with a thermodilution-based catheter. The mean catheter-right ventricular ejection fraction was 41±9% and the mean fractional area change by on-line echocardiography was 40±8% with significant correlation between the two methods (r=0.74).

Applications During Intraoperative Monitoring

The first study that employed on-line measurements of left LV areas and fractional area change in the operating room with the use of transesophageal imaging was published by Cahalan and coworkers. [59] They studied 25 patients monitored by transesophageal imaging before cardiac surgery (Figure 3.16). In their experience, the border-detection on-line method underestimated the off-line determined fractional area change in short axis images (0.44±0.03% vs. 0.56±0.03%). However the authors employed separate set of images for comparison (not the same cardiac cycle analyzed simultaneously, as previously discussed). In addition, the study was carried out without the benefits of lateral gain compensation (not available in the early versions of the system) which may have contributed to the relatively poor correlations.

Figure 3.16. Top: plot of all area measurements from automated border detection (ABD) versus conventional laboratory analysis (LAB). End-diastolic data pairs (EDA) are shown as closed triangles, and end-systolic data pairs (ESA) as open circles (n = 25 for each). Correlations were r=0.975 for EDA with SE of 1.18 cm² and r=0.937 for ESA with SE of 1.17 cm². The two solid diagonal

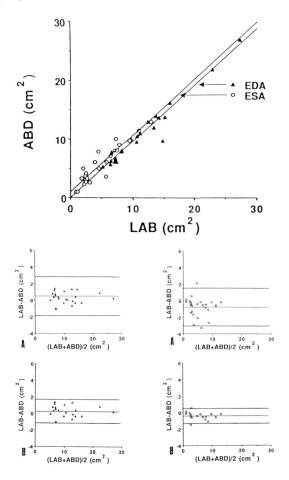

lines are the lines for best fit for the EDA and ESA data as indicated by the arrows. Bottom left panels: bias analysis for all end-diastolic area (n=25). For each data pair, the difference between the laboratory estimate (LAB) and the automatic border detection (ABD) estimate of the EDA is plotted versus the mean of the measurements. The middle solid line indicates the average difference between the LAB and ABD estimates or the bias. The outer (upper and lower) heavy solid lines indicate two standard deviations of the mean differences and define the limits of the agreement. Approximately 95% of the differences lie within the limits of the agreement. All data is expressed in cm². Bottom right panels: bias analysis of all end-systolic area (ESA) data (n=25) with explanations identical to that of left panels. (Reproduced with permission from Cahalan *et al.*, *Anesthesiology* 1993;78:477-485).

In another study where on-line measurements of LV cavity area and fractional area change were compared to off-line manual tracing of the images, Perrino *et al.* [60] studied 18 patients by transesophageal echocardiography during anesthesia preceding cardiac surgery. Adequate short axis images were obtained in 72% of patients (short axis) and only in 5 patients (28%) in the longitudinal view. A comparison of 122 matched segments yielded a high correlation (r=0.96) between on-line diastolic areas and off-line traced images. The correlation for end-systolic areas and fractional area change were 0.97 and 0.86, respectively, with the on-line measurements exhibiting an underestimation of the off-line areas in diastole and systole and of the fractional area change.

Application for Assessment of the Right Ventricle

Recently, studies by Rassmussen *et al.* [61] have demonstrated the utility of the on-line measurement system for the evaluation of the right ventricular cavity area and fractional area change in 20 patients with pulmonary hypertension before and after pulmonary thromboendarterectomy. The mean values of end-diastolic, end-systolic right ventricular cavity areas and fractional area change correlated rather poorly with those obtained by off-line traced areas (r=0.39, 0.41 and 0.45). These results are not surprising after considering the more complex shape of the right ventricle (as compared to that of the left ventricle), the influence of the presence of the moderator band upon the on-line vs. off-line planimetered cavity areas, the analysis of non-simultaneous beats and the relative difficulty in visualizing the right ventricular apical region in all patients.

Conclusions

The introduction of an objective, rapid and reliable method of obtaining measurements of cardiac chamber area and estimated volumes on-line by echocardiography has caused a renewal in the efforts to obtain precise quantification of cardiac chamber dimensions and function illustrated by the variety of applications and validation studies carried out with this technique worldwide in a relatively short time. Validation studies of a new technique against existing methodologies is always an important exercise that must be undertaken with fair and comparable data sets. In this case, the use of simultaneous paired data (the same cardiac cycle analyzed by both approaches) seems the most appropriate as has been carried out in several of the studies. In addition, such type of analysis must be accompanied by bias analysis to ascertain the validity of the application. Despite the disparate approach, information and knowledge gained by multiple investigators, and the various experimental and clinical conditions in which it has been employed, the method yields acceptable results. The technique of performing on-line quantification of ventricular dimensions and function has been, and continues to be, extensively studied in order to place it in the proper perspective of the practice of echocardiography in the future. At the least, its introduction has awaken the interest in quantification of two-dimensional images at a time when those involved in the practice of echocardiography are required to demonstrate quality, efficacy and efficiency in our daily workload.

References

1. Feigenbaum H. Evolution of echocardiography. *Circulation* 1996;93:1321-7.
2. Sahn DJ, DeMaria A, Kisslo J, Weyman A: Recommendations regarding quantitation in M-Mode echocardiography: Results of a survey of echocardiographic measurements. *Circulation* 1978; 58:1072-1080.
3. Katz AS, Force TL, Folland ED, Aebischer N, Sharma S, Parisi AF: Echocardiographic assessment of ventricular systolic function. In: Skorton DJ, Schelbert HR, Wolf GL, and Brundage BH eds. *Marcus Cardiac Imaging: A Companion to Braunwald's Heart Disease.* Philadelphia, PA, Saunders, 1996; I:297-324
4. Gopal AS, Shen Z, Sapin PM, Keller AM, Schnellbaecher MJ, Leibowitz DW, Akinboboye OO, Rodney RA, Blood DK, King DL: Assessment of cardiac function by three-dimensional echocardiography compared with conventional noninvasive methods. *Circulation* 1995;92:842-853.
5. Schiller NB, Shah PM, Crawford M, DeMaria A, Devereaux R, Feigenbaum H, Gutgesell H, Reichek N, Sahn D, Schnittger I: Recommendations for quantitation of the left ventricle by two-dimensional echocardiography. *J Am Soc Echocardiogr* 1989;2:358-367.
6. Skorton DJ, McNary CA, Child JS, Newton FC, Shah PM: Digital image processing of two dimensional echocardiograms: Identification of the endocardium. *Am J Cardiol* 1981;48:479-486.
7. Zwehl W, Levy R, Garcia E, Haendchen RV, Childs W, Corday SR, Meerbaum S, Corday E: Validation of a computerized edge detection algorithm for quantitative two dimensional echocardiography. *Circulation* 1983;64:1127-1135.
8. Collins SM, Skorton DJ, Geiser EA, Nicholas JA, Conetta DA, Pandian NG, Kerber RE: Computer-assisted edge detection in the two dimensional echocardiography: Comparison with anatomic data. *Am J Cardiol* 1984;S3:1380-1387.

9. Geiser EA, Wilson DC, Gibby GL, Billett J, Conetta DA: A method for evaluation of enhancement operations in two dimensional echocardiographic images. *J Am Soc Echocardiogr* 1991;4:235-246.

10. Chu CH, Delp EJ, Buda AJ: Detecting left ventricular endocardial and epicardial boundaries by digital two dimensional echocardiography. *IEEE Trans Med Imaging* 1988;7:81-90.

11. Friedland N, Adam D: Automatic ventricular cavity boundary detection from sequential ultrasound images using simulated annealing. *IEEE Trans Med Imaging* 1989;8:344-353.

12. Geiser EA, Oliver CH, Gardin JM, Kerber RE, Parisi A, Reichek N, Werner JA, Weyman AE: Clinical validation of an edge detection algorithm for two dimensional echocardiographic short axis images. *J Am Soc Echocardiogr* 1988;1:410-421.

13. Geiser EA, Wilson DJ, Gibby GL: A second generation computer edge detection algorithm for short axis two dimensional echocardiographic images, accuracy and improvement in interobserver variability. *J Am Soc Echocardiogr* 1990;3:79-90.

14. Pérez JE, Holland MR, Barzilai B, Handley SM, Vandenberg B, Miller JG, Skorton DJ: Ultrasonic characterization of cardiovascular tissue. In: Skorton DJ, Schelbert HR, Wolf GL, and Brundage BH eds. *Marcus Cardiac Imaging: A Companion to Braunwald's Heart Disease*. Philadelphia, PA, Saunders, 1996;I:606-627.

15. Pérez JE, Waggoner AD, Barzilai B, Melton HE, Miller JG, Sobel BE: New edge detection algorithm facilitates two dimensional echocardiographic on-line analysis of left ventricular performance. *J Am Coll Cardiol* 1991;17:291A (Abstract)..

16. Vandenberg BF, Rathl L, Stuhlmuller P, Melton HE, Skorton DJ: Estimation of left ventricular cavity area with a new on-line automated echocardiographic edge detection system. *J Am Coll Cardiol* 1991;17:291A (Abstract).

17. Melton HE, Collins SM, Skorton DJ: Automatic real-time endocardial edge detection in two-dimensional echocardiography. *Ultrasound Imaging* 1983;5:300-307.

18. Bednarz JF, Marcus RH, Lang RM: Technical guidelines for performing automated border detection studies. *J Am Soc Echocardiogr* 1995;8:293-305.

19. Pérez JE, Waggoner AD, Barzilai B, Melton HE, Jr., Miller JG, Sobel BE: On-line assessment of ventricular function by automatic boundary detection and ultrasonic backscatter imaging. *J Am Coll Cardiol* 1992;19:313-320.

20. Vandenberg BF, Rath LS, Stuhlmuller RN, Melton HE, Skorton DJ: Estimation of left ventricular cavity area with an on-line, semiautomated echocardiographic edge detection system. *Circulation* 1992;86:159-166.

21. Vandenberg B, Cardona H, Miller JG, Skorton DJ, Pérez JE: On-line left ventricular volume measurement in patients using automated border detection: Comparison with conventional echocardiography. *Circulation* 1992;86:I-262 (Abstract).

22. Mugge A, Daniel WG, Grote J, Hausmann D, Niedemyer J, Lichtlen PR: Acoustic quantification - a new on-line automated echocardiographic edge detection system for continuous analysis of left ventricular areas and function. *Eur Heart J* 1992;13:316 (Astract).

23. Herregods MC, Vermylen J, Bynens B, DeGeest H, Van De Werf F: On-line quantification of left ventricular function by automatic boundary detection and ultrasonic backscatter imaging. *Am J Cardiol* 1993;72:359-362.

24. Cao QL, Ramadurai M, Hsu TL, Pandian N: Factors influencing real-time automated border detection and acoustic quantification and practical tips for optimal analysis of ventricular function. *J Am Soc Echocardiogr* 1992;5:335 (Abstract).

25. Cao QL, Azevedo J, Hsu TL, Pandian N: Real-time automated border detection and acoustic quantification in biplane and multiplane transesophageal echocardiography and factors influencing its accuracy. *Circulation* 1992;86:I-263 (Abstract).

26. Torrecilla EG, Garcia-Fernandez MA, San Roman D, Bueno H, Valero R, Delcan JL: Echocardiographic automated border detection: Transthoracic versus transesophageal approaches. *Eur Heart J* 1992;13:316 (Abstract).

27. Stoddard MF, Keedy DL: Acoustical quantification of left ventricular area is highly feasible during transesophageal echocardiography. *J Am Coll Cardiol* 1993;21:84A (Abstract).

28. Dávila-Román VG, Cardona H, Feinberg M, Pérez JE, Barzilai B: Quantification of left ventricular dimensions on line with biplane transesophageal echocardiography and lateral gain compensation. *Echocardiography* 1994;11:119-125.

29. Lindower PD, Rath L, Preslar J, Burns T, Rezai K, Vandenberg B: Acoustic quantification of left ventricular function: Comparison with isotope ventriculography. *J Am Soc Echo* 1992;5:335 (Abstract).

30. San Roman D, Garcia-Fernandez MA, Torrecilla EG, Dominquez P, Bittini A, Bueno H. Delcan JL: Left ventricular function assessment by automatic border detection echocardiography. Radionuclide ventriculography validation. *Eur Heart J* 1992;13:316 (Absract).

31. Cao QL, Azevedo J, Snapper H, Schwartz S, Udelson J, Pandian N: Automated, on-line determination of left ventricular volumes and ejection fraction by acoustic quantification: (1) *in vitro* validation, (2) *in vivo* comparison with radionuclide method in patients, (3) examination of factors influencing its accuracy, and (4) clinical application. *J Am Coll Cardiol* 1993;21:275A (Abstract).

32. Gorcsan J III, Lazar JM, Schulman DS, Follansbee WP: Comparison of left ventricular function by echocardiographic automated border detection and by radionuclide ejection fraction. *Am J Cardiol* 1993;72:810-815.

33. Lindower PD, Rath L, Preslar J, Burns TL, Rezai K, Vandenberg BF: Quantification of left ventricular function with an automated border detection system and comparison with radionuclide ventriculography. *Am J Cardiol* 1994;73:195-199.

34. Yvorchuk KJ, Davies RA, Chan KL: Measurement of left ventricular ejection fraction by acoustic quantification and comparison with radionuclide angiography. *Am J Cardiol* 1994;74:1052-1056.

35. Epperlein S, Wittlich N, Erbel R, Trautmann S, Meyer J: Acoustic quantification--on-line assessment of left ventricular function by real-time automatic, boundary detection in two-dimensional echocardiography. *Eur Heart J* 1993;14:68.

36. Vanoverschelde JJ, Hanet C, Wijns W, Detry JM: On-line quantification of left ventricular volumes and ejection fraction by automated backscatter imaging-assisted

boundary detection: Comparison with contrast cineventriuclography. *Am J Cardiol* 1994;74:633-635.

37. Marcus RH, Bednarz J, Coulden R, Shroff S, Lipton M, Lang RM: Ultrasonic backscatter system for automated on-line endocardial boundary detection: Evaluation by ultrafast computed tomography. *J Am Coll Cardiol* 1993;29:839-847.

38. Stewart WJ, Rodkey SM, Gutawardena S, White RD, Luvisi B, Klein AL, Salcedo E: Left ventricular volume calculation with integrated backscatter from echocardiography. *J Am Soc Echocardiogr* 1993;6:553-563.

39. Gorcsan J III, Lazar JM, Romand J, Pinsky MR: On-line estimation of stroke volume by means of echocardiographic automated border detection in the canine left ventricle. *Am Heart J* 1993;125:1316-1323.

40. Morrissey RL, Siu SC, Guerrero JL, Weyman AB, Picard MH: Ventricular volume by echocardiographic automated border detection: On-line calculation without loss of accuracy. *J Am Coll Cardiol* 1993;21:275A (Abstract).

41. Azevedo J, Cao QL, Schwartz S, Pandian N: Novel combination of automated acoustic quantification and 3-dimensional reconstruction for quantitative and qualitative evaluation of the size, geometry, volume and function of left ventricular aneurysms-experimental and clinical studies. *J Am Soc Echocardiogr* 1993;6:S7 (Abstract).

42. Jiang L, Morrissey R, Handschumacher MD, He J, Picard MH, Weyman AE, Levine RA: Can acoustic quantification be applied on three dimensional echocardiographic resolution? *Circulation* 1993;88:I-161 (Abstract).

43. Morrissey RL, Siu SC, Guerrero JL, Newell JB, Weyman AE, Picard MH: Automated assessment of ventricular volume and function by echocardiography: validation of automated border detection. *J Am Soc Echocardiogr* 1994;7:107-115.

44. Paulsen PR, Pavek T, Crampton M, Herrliger S, Homans DC: Validation of automatic edge detection echocardiography: Assessment of rate of LV cavity expansion and contraction. *Circulation* 1992;86:I-262 (Abstract).

45. Pérez JE, Klein SC, Prater DM, Fraser CE, Cardona H, Waggoner AD, Holland MR, Miller JG, Sobel BE: On-line quantification of left ventricular dimensions and function by echocardiography with backscatter imaging and lateral gain compensation. *Am J Cardiol* 1992;70:1200-1205.

46. Tutt LK, Lopelen HA, Vukovic HS, Soto JG, Zoghbi WA, Quinones MA: Acoustic quantification of fractional area change of the left ventricle: Reproducibility of results between technologists in a non-selected cardiac population. *Circulation* 1992;86:I-264 (Abstract)..

47. Waggoner AD, Miller JG, Pérez JE: Two dimensional echocardiographic automatic boundary detection for evaluation of left ventricular function in unselected adult patients. *J Am Soc Echo* 1994;7:459-464.

48. Seliem MA, McWilliams ET, Palileo M: Beat-to-beat variability of left ventricular indexes measured by acoustic quantification: influence of heart rate and respiration-correlation with M-Mode echocardiography. *J Am Soc Echocardiogr* 1996;9:221-230.

49. Pinto FJ, Siegel LC, Kreitzmann TR, Davidson R, Popp RL, Schnittger I: On-line estimation of cardiac output with a new automated edge detection system using transesophageal echocardiography: Comparison with thermodilution. *Circulation* 1991;84:II-585 (Abstract).

50. Tardif JC, Cao QL, Pandian NG, Esakof DD, Pollard H: Determination of cardiac output using acoustic quantification in critically ill patients. *Am J Cardiol* 1994;74:810-813.

51. Feinberg MS, Davila-Roman VG, Hopkins WE, Spray TL, Perez JE, Barzilai B: Successful withdrawal of biventricular assist devices after assessment of left ventricular function by transesophageal echocardiography and automatic border detection. *Echocardiography* 1994;11:575-578.

52. Sun JP, Stewart WJ, Yang XS, Lee KS, Sheldon WS, Thomas JD: Automated echocardiographic quantification of left ventricular volumes and ejection fraction; validation in the intensive care setting. . *J Am Soc Echocardiogr* 1995;8:29-36.

53. Dávila-Román VG, Creswell LL, Rosenbloom M, Pérez JE: Myocardial conytractile state in dogs with chronic mitral regurgitation: Echocardiographic approach to the peak systolic pressure end-systolic area relationship. *Am Heart J* 1993;126:155-160.

54. Iliceto S, Pellegrini C, Napoli F, Caiati C, Manangelli V, Memmola C, Rizzon P: Automatic evaluation of stress-induced left ventricular area changes with a new on-line echocardiographic edge detection system. *Circulation* 1991;84:II-585 (Abstract).

55. Pérez JE, Waggoner AD, Dávila-Román VG, Cardona H, Miller JG: On-line quantification of ventricular function during dobutamine stress echocardiography. *Eur Heart J* 1992;13:1669-1676.

56. Dubourg O, Jondeau G, Dib JC, Chikli F, Beauchet A, Guertet P, Bourdarias JP: Value of an automated border detection system for studying left ventricular diastolic and systolic function in normal subjects. *Eur Heart J* 1992;13:317 (Abstract).

57. San Roman D, Garcia-Fernandez MA, Torrecilla EG, Ixcamparij C, Gutierrez A, Gonzalez A, Rico M, Delcan JL: On-line estimation of left ventricular function using automatic border detection from intracardiac echocardiography. *Eur Heart J* 1992;13:317 (Abstract).

58. Schneider A, Schwartz S, Pandian N, Gordon G, England M, Warner K: Utility of on-line automated acoustic quantification in the evaluation of right ventricular function: Comparison with rapid response thermistor catheter measurement of right ventricular ejection fraction. *J Am Coll Cardiol* 1993;21

59. Cahalan MK, Ionescu P, Melton HE, Adler S, Kee LL, Schiller NB: Automated real-time analysis of intraoperative transesophageal echocardiograms. *Anesthesiology* 1993;78:477-485.

60. Perrino AC Jr., Luther MA, O'Connor TZ, Cohen IS: Automated border detection: odd-line validation of serial intraoperative measurements. *Anesthesiology* 1994;81:3A (Abstract)

61. Rassmussen CM, Dyer D, Wheeler K, Donaghey L, Kwan OL, Dittrich HC: Automatic border detection to assess right ventricular function following surgical treatment of thromboembolic pulmonary hypertension. *Echocardiography* 1996;13:109-116.

4 Automated Assessment of Left Ventricular Function with Acoustic Quantification: Signal Averaging Revisited

Victor Mor-Avi, James E. Bednarz,
Kirk T. Spencer, Philippe Vignon,
Amy C. Bales, and Roberto M. Lang

Why Signal Averaging?

Acoustic quantification (AQ) allows continuous real-time measurements of the cross-sectional area of the heart chambers by differentiating the acoustic backscatter characteristics of blood from those of myocardial tissue within an operator defined region of interest [1,2]. By providing on-line beat-to-beat information on clinically important physiologic parameters, this technology facilitates quantitative non-invasive assessment of hemodynamic responses to pharmacological and surgical interventions [3-5].

Although many studies have consistently endorsed the AQ technology, a critical review of the literature reveals that most validation studies used manually selected single AQ waveforms for comparison with other techniques [6-10]. The need for manual selection of beats arose from the fact that AQ signals are frequently noisy and accordingly suffer from significant inter-beat variability [11] (Figure 4.1). Moreover, their time-derivatives, which are required to characterize diastolic dysfunction, are often uninterpretable due to noise (Figure 4.2, left), which may result from a variety of factors such as poor endocardial tracking, intrinsic cardiac translation and/or rotation, or even a minimal movement of the patient or sonographer [3,11]. Additionally, respiratory variations which originate from physiologic cardiac volume changes are commonly observed in AQ signals in normal subjects and are accentuated in patients with dyspnea. The inter-beat variability in AQ waveforms may have a negative impact on the reproducibility of the estimated parameters of cardiac function by altering the imaging plane relative to the position of the region of interest and impairing the detection of the endocardial boundary.

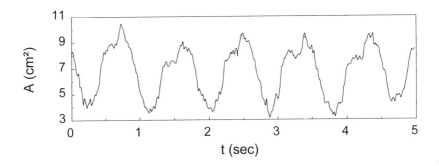

Figure 4.1. Left ventricular area signal obtained from a short-axis view at the papillary muscle level using acoustic quantification technology. Note the noise and large interbeat variability.

Since most of these technical limitations and physiologic variables are difficult to eliminate, we hypothesized that signal averaging of multiple AQ waveforms could minimize the beat to beat variability and thus enhance the accuracy and clinical utility of this technique. In particular, its ability to assess LV diastolic function, which heavily relies on the quality of the time-derivatives of AQ waveforms, would be improved. Accordingly, we developed a software for signal averaging of AQ waveforms, based on principles which have been previously utilized extensively in electrocardiography to reduce noise and unmask important morphological details [12]. Our fully automated algorithm is based on a computer-determined template waveform which is used for automated serial beat detection, accurate temporal alignment of beats, and rejection of beats which are morphologically different from the template beyond a preset threshold [13]. Even though the computer-made choice of template has to be confirmed by the operator and the similarity threshold for averaging may vary, we found that in normal subjects, the effects of selecting different templates or thresholds on the values of the different indices of LV function are insignificant [13]. Prior to presenting examples describing the clinical utility of this software it is necessary to describe the morphology, parameters and physiologic correlates of normal left ventricular and left atrial waveforms.

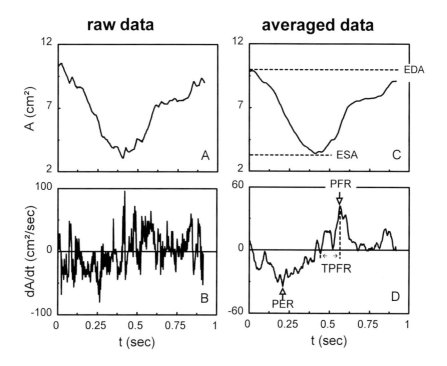

Figure 4.2. Representative raw data waveform and its time derivative (left upper and lower panels, respectively). Note the high level of noise which hampers accurate evaluation of LV function. After signal averaging, the reduction in noise is easily appreciated when comparing the average waveform with single beat data (right upper and lower panels, respectively). The high amplitude of noise observed in the time derivative is eliminated by signal averaging. As a result, end-diastolic and end-systolic area (EDA, ESA), peak ejection and peak filling rates (PER and PFR), as well as the time to peak filling rate (TPFR) can be easily identified. (Please note the difference in scale between the two lower panels).

Normal Waveforms, Derived Parameters and Physiologic Correlates

LV Volume Measurements

Acoustic quantification offers two different geometric and mathematical models for the calculation of LV volume from an apical view described in Chapter 1. Figure 4.3 presents an example of a signal averaged LV volume waveform and its time derivative, wherein the three different phases of LV filling, namely rapid filling, conduit phase and atrial contraction, can be easily identified.

Ejection Fraction

Ejection fraction is calculated as the left ventricular stroke volume normalized to the end-diastolic volume (Table 4.1). This commonly used ejection phase index reflects the net interaction between cardiac loading conditions (i.e., preload, afterload and heart rate) and contractile state [14,15].

Rate of Volume Change, Peak Filling and Ejection Rates and Time to Peak Filling Rate

The instantaneous rate of volume change throughout the cardiac cycle is calculated as follows:

$$\frac{dV}{dt} = \frac{Volume_{frame_n} - Volume_{frame_{n-1}}}{Time_{frame_n} - Time_{frame_{n-1}}}$$

The peak filling rate (PFR) measures the peak rate of LV volume increase during ventricular diastole. The PFR can be expressed as a fraction of the end-diastolic volume per second. The time to peak filling rate (TPFR) is measured as the time interval between end-systole (minimum LV volume) and the occurrence of peak filling rate (Table 4.1). The values of PFR and TPFR have been previously determined using radionuclide techniques in patients with coronary artery disease, hypertrophic cardiomyopathy, and hypertensive heart disease [16-23]. Although correlations between abnormalities of diastolic function and these AQ-derived indices have been reported [7,8], both PFR and TPFR are dependent on ventricular loading conditions, heart rate, contractility and systolic performance. The method for adjusting these indices for ventricular size and function remains controversial. While normalization by end-diastolic volume improves the clinical utility of these indices, they nevertheless reflect the interactive nature of the multiple variables that characterize the complex physiology of diastole.

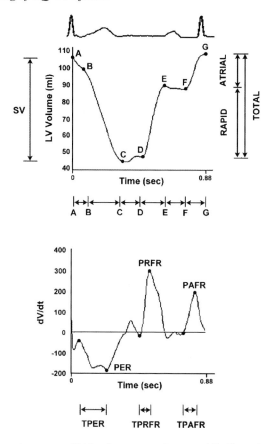

Figure 4.3. Signal averaged LV volume waveform and its time derivative (dV/dt). A-B, isovolumic contraction; B-C, ventricular ejection; C-D, isovolumic relaxation; D-E, rapid diastolic filling; E-F, diastasis; F-G, filling secondary to atrial contraction; SV, stroke volume; PER, peak ejection rate; PRFR, peak rapid filling rate; PAFR, peak atrial filling rate; TPER, time to peak ejection rate; TPRFR, time to peak rapid filling rate; TPAFR, time to peak atrial filling rate. During systole, LV volume decreases from its highest value at end-diastole (A) to its lowest value at end-systole (C). The difference between end-diastolic and end-systolic volume represents total LV stroke volume (SV). Following the end-of-ejection, the period of isovolumic relaxation starts and intraventricular pressure rapidly falls below left atrial pressure levels. LV volume increases during early rapid diastolic filling and is followed by a period of diastasis (E-F) during which only minimal changes in LV volume occur. During the latter third of diastole, left atrial contraction ejects an additional bolus of blood into the left ventricle; atrial systole accounts for approximately 20% to 30% of LV filling in normal hearts.

Table 4.1. Formulas used for AQ-based measurements. (*Reprinted with permission from J Am Soc Echocardiogr 1995;8:293-305*)

AQ measurement	Formula	Normal values
EDV end-diastolic volume	$$V_{MOD} = \frac{n\pi}{4L} \sum_{i=1}^{n} A_i^2$$	89-133 ml
ESV end-systolic volume	$$V_{AL} = \frac{8A^2}{3\pi L}$$	23-45 ml
EF ejection fraction	$$\frac{EDV - ESV}{EDV} * 100$$	50-80%
PFR peak filling rate (normalized)	$$\frac{\left(\frac{dV}{dt}\right)_{max}}{EDV}$$	2.0-4.5 EDV/sec
PER peak ejection rate (normalized)	$$\frac{\left(\frac{dV}{dt}\right)_{min}}{EDV}$$	1.7-4.0 EDV/sec
TPFR time to peak filling rate	$$TIME_{\left(\frac{dV}{dt}\right)_{max}} - TIME_{ESV}$$	110-230 msec

V_{MOD} - method of discs volume, V_{AL} - area-length method volume, n - the number of discs, L - LV length, A_i - area of a disc, A - LV area, ESV and EDV - end-systolic and end-diastolic volume, $(dV/dt)_{max}$ - maximum volume derivative, $(dV/dt)_{min}$ - minimum volume derivative.

Two issues must be addressed to determine the clinical utility of TPFR obtained with AQ: (1) TPFR cannot be defined more precisely than the variable frame rate delay, and (2) TPFR assumes that the minimum of the AQ waveform corresponds to end-systole. Since minimum volume may occur early in diastole due to cardiac rotation or translation during isovolumic relaxation, TPFR determined without signal averaging should be interpreted with caution.

The peak ejection rate, an index of systolic performance, is calculated as the minimal value of the first derivative of LV volume, and may also be normalized by end-diastolic volume. Similar to all ejection phase indices, it is load and heart rate dependent [14,15]. The normal ranges in Table 4.1 were obtained using radionuclide imaging. Normal values for these parameters when obtained with AQ and their age and gender dependence have yet to be established.

Left Atrial Area Measurements

Left atrial AQ area waveforms can aid in the ʹassessment of the mechanical function of the left atrium. Figure 4.4 depicts an example of a signal averaged left atrial area waveform and its time derivative. During ventricular systole, the left atrium fills via the pulmonic veins. During ventricular diastole, the left atrium empties in three distinct phases: (1) passive emptying which coincides with rapid ventricular filling, (2) diastasis or conduit phase, and (3) active emptying which coincides with atrial systole. As described in Chapter 7, echocardiographic evaluation of left atrial function is limited, and normal values for left atrial filling and emptying have not been well established [24-26].

Clinical Applications of Signal Averaged AQ Waveforms

We first tested the clinical feasibility of using signal averaging of AQ waveforms to assess LV diastolic function in patients with dilated cardiomyopathy and hypertensive subjects with concentric left ventricular hypertrophy and normal sinus rhythm. Subsequently, the averaging algorithm was used to assess pharmacologically induced alterations in LV function. Finally, we studied the feasibility of repeated analysis of signal averaged AQ waveforms obtained with transesophageal echocardiography as a tool for long-term monitoring of LV function in the intensive care unit setting.

Signal averaged LV volume waveforms were obtained in 12 patients with dilated cardiomyopathy and 12 age-matched normal subjects. As expected, patients with dilated cardiomyopathy had increased end-diastolic and end-systolic volumes with reduced ejection fractions [27] (Figure 4.5). From the signal averaged LV volume waveforms it was possible to calculate both peak ejection and filling rates as well as the time to peak filling rate, which were significantly different compared to the normal group (Table 4.2).

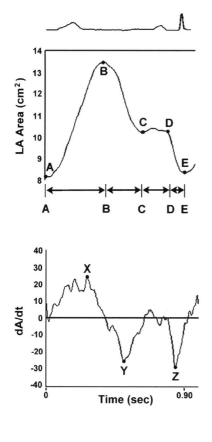

Figure 4.4. Signal averaged left atrial area waveform and its time derivative. A-B, left atrial filling occurring during ventricular systole; B-C, passive emptying of the left atrium into the LV coinciding with rapid ventricular filling phase; C-D, left atrial diastasis; D-E, active emptying due to left atrial contraction; X, corresponds to the peak rate of atrial filling; Y, the peak rate of left atrial passive emptying; Z, the peak rate of left atrial active emptying.

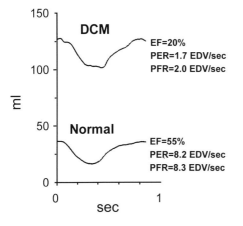

Figure 4.5. Signal averaged LV volume curves obtained in a patient with a dilated cardiomyopathy (DCM) and in an age-matched normal subject. In addition to the obvious differences in LV dimensions between subjects, please note the presence of systolic and diastolic dysfunction quantitated in terms of reduced peak ejection and peak filling rates (PER and PFR), respectively.

Table 4.2. Parameters of LV function obtained from signal averaged LV volume waveforms in 12 patients with dilated cardiomyopathy (DCM) and 12 age matched normal (NL) subjects. (*p<0.01).

	Age	EDV(ml)	ESV(ml)	EF(%)	PFR(EDV/s)	PER(EDV/s)	tPFR(RR)
NL	44±4	61±21	35±17	44±10	4.6±1.6	4.9±2.0	0.10±0.04
DCM	49±8	130±47*	105±46*	21±9*	1.8±0.9*	2.1±1.4*	0.17±0.08*

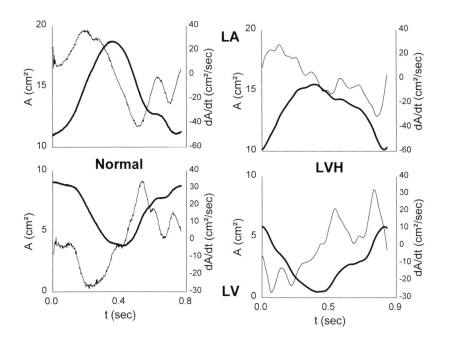

Figure 4.6. Signal averaged left ventricular and left atrial area waveforms and their time derivatives obtained in a patient with left ventricular hypertrophy (LVH) and in an age matched normal subject. In the patient with LVH, augmented LV filling occurs during late diastole, reflecting increased contribution of left atrial contraction towards LV filling. These changes are also evidenced in the left atrial waveforms which demonstrate augmented active versus passive emptying.

In patients with concentric left ventricular hypertrophy this methodology was able to demonstrate augmented contribution of atrial contraction towards LV filling [7,8]. Signal averaged waveforms reflecting left ventricular and left atrial cross-sectional area were obtained in 33 patients with LV hypertrophy, and in age matched normal subjects. Both left ventricular and left atrial waveforms had markedly different morphology in patients with left ventricular hypertrophy, compared to normal controls (Figure 4.6). Left ventricular waveforms were used to calculate indices of LV diastolic function such as: PFR, (t)PFR, $F_{1/3}FF$ (first third filling fraction), and AFF (atrial filling fraction). Left atrial area waveforms were also averaged to assess left atrial performance by calculating $F_{1/3}EF$ (first third emptying fraction). Patients with LV hypertrophy had lower PFR, $F_{1/3}FF$ and higher AFF consistent with abnormal LV relaxation (Table 4.3). In addition, left atrial $F_{1/3}EF$ was reduced compared to the control group.

Table 4.3: Parameters of diastolic function obtained from signal averaged LV area waveforms in 33 patients with left ventricular hypertrophy (LVH) and 33 normal (NL) subjects. (*$p<0.05$).

	Age	LV mass (g)	PFR(EDA/s)	tPFR(msec)	F1/3FF(%)	AFF(%)
NL	59±14	133±36	5.1±1.2	60±29	58±12	27±10
LVH	58±14	306±110*	4.2±1.3*	69±40	49±15*	35±15*

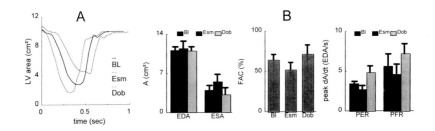

Figure 4.7. (A) Example of signal averaged LV area waveforms obtained in a normal subject under baseline conditions (BL), and during infusions of esmolol (Esm) and dobutamine (Dob). he end-systolic area decreased with dobutamine and increased with esmolol. (B) Summary of LV function parameters (A = LV area, FAC = fractional area change, peak dA/dt (EDA/s) = peak filling rate) obtained in 8 normal subjects under baseline conditions, and during infusions of esmolol and dobutamine.

To further investigate the ability of AQ enhanced by signal averaging to assess LV systolic and diastolic function, we acquired and analyzed data in 8 normal subjects (age 31±4) under baseline conditions and during intravenous infusions of esmolol and dobutamine [28]. In all subjects, signal averaged AQ area waveforms clearly demonstrated the expected alterations in LV function caused by these agents. When compared to control conditions, the slope of the initial portion of the descending and ascending limb of the LV area waveforms decreased with esmolol and increased with dobutamine (Figure 4.7,A). Left ventricular systolic fractional area change (FAC) and diastolic filling fraction (FF) and peak ejection and filling rates decreased with esmolol and increased with dobutamine (Figure 4.7,B). These results provided additional support to the hypothesis that AQ in conjunction with signal averaging constitutes a sensitive tool capable of tracking even subtle variations in LV diastolic function (see Chapter 5).

The results of these studies suggested that continuous acquisition and signal averaging of AQ waveforms with repeated analysis may allow noninvasive monitoring of LV function [29]. We modified our signal averaging software accordingly, so that the average waveform of the current averaging cycle is used as the template for the subsequent cycle (Figure 4.8). This allowed us to perform repeated signal averaging for long periods of time without the need for further intervention.

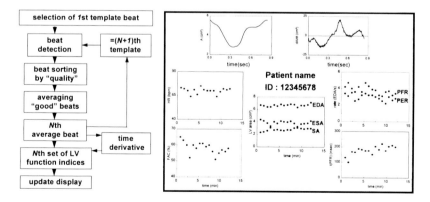

Figure 4.8. Flow chart describing repeated signal averaging procedure used for continuous monitoring of LV function (left). Typical display of the monitoring system after 12 minutes of continuous monitoring (right).

We hypothesized that when combined with transesophageal imaging, which provides excellent imaging quality and stable images, this approach would allow objective display of LV hemodynamic trends reflecting the rapid changes that occur in the intensive care or operating room setting. To test this hypothesis, LV area signals were obtained and repeatedly averaged for 1 to 2 hours in 7 patients undergoing abdominal surgery [29]. The measured values of end-systolic and end-diastolic area and fractional area change were displayed as a function of time and compared with simultaneously acquired invasive data (Figure 4.9). This monitoring system facilitated early recognition of hypovolemic and cardiac dysfunction episodes, and accurately tracked hemodynamic changes resulting from therapeutic interventions. In all cases, the invasive hemodynamic data correlated closely with the information provided by trasnesophageal echocardiographic monitoring. Accordingly, it appears that continuous signal averaging of AQ waveforms in the operating room is feasible and allows reliable long-term monitoring of LV function in real time.

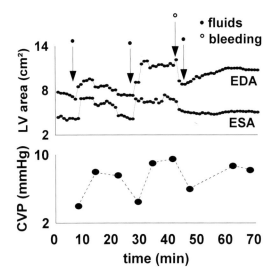

Figure 4.9. Example of hemodynamic data obtained in a patient undergoing abdominal surgery using the noninvasive monitoring system based on AQ (top) compared with simultaneously measured central venous pressures (CVP). Note the close correlation between invasive and noninvasive data. Arrows represent intraoperative bleeding episodes which resulted in a decrease in LV area .

Summary

In summary, Acoustic Quantification allows real-time automated endocardial boundary detection which is vital for on-line measurement of LV dimensions. In conjunction with signal averaging, this noninvasive technique allows fast, easy and accurate quantification of LV systolic and diastolic performance. This technique is sensitive enough to track even minute-by-minute trends in multiple indices of LV function. It has great clinical potential as a tool to assess LV function in different disease states, as well as a guide to select the most efficient therapeutic interventions.

Acknowledgement

We wish to thank the sonographers at the University of Chicago Noninvasive Cardiac Imaging Laboratories for their contributions.

References

1. Perez JE, Klein SC, Prater DM, Fraser CE, Cardona H, Waggoner AD, Holland MR, Miller JG, Sobel BE: Automated, on-line quantification of left ventricular dimensions and function by echocardiography with backscatter imaging and lateral gain compensation. *Am J Cardiol* 1992;70:1200-1205.
2. Perez JE, Waggoner AD, Barzilai B, Melton HE, Miller JG, Sobel BE: On-line assessment of ventricular function by automatic boundary detection and ultrasonic backscatter imaging. *J Am Coll Cardiol* 1992;19:313-320.
3. Perez JE, Waggoner AD, Davila-Roman VD, Cardona H, Miller JG: On-line quantification of ventricular function during dobutamine stress echocardiography. *Eur Heart J* 1992;13:1669-1676.
4. Gorcsan J, 3d, Gasior TA, Mandarino WA, Deneault LG, Hattler BG, Pinsky MR: On-line estimation of changes in left ventricular stroke volume by transesophageal echocardiographic automated border detection in patients undergoing coronary artery bypass grafting. *Am J Cardiol* 1993;72:721-727.
5. Gorcsan J, 3d, Lazar JM, Schulman DS, Follansbee WP: Comparison of left ventricular function by echocardiographic automated border detection and by radionuclide ejection fraction. *Am J Cardiol* 1993;72:810-815.
6. Marcus RH, Bednarz JE, Coulden R, Shroff S, Lipton M, Lang RM: Ultrasonic backscatter system for automated on-line endocardial boundary detection: evaluation by ultrafast computed tomography. *J Am Coll Cardiol* 1993;22:839-847.

7. Chenzbraun A, Pinto FJ, Popylisen S, Schnittger I, Popp RI: Filling patterns in left ventricular hypertrophy: a combined acoustic quantification and Doppler study. *J Am Col Cardiol* 1994;23:1179-1185.

8. Chenzbraun A, Pinto FJ, Popylisen S, Schnittger I, Popp RL: Comparison of acoustic quantification and Doppler echocardiography in assessment of left ventricular variables. *Br Heart J* 1993;70:448-456.

9. Lang RM, Bednarz J, Weinert L, Balasia B, Korcarz C, Marcus R: End-systolic pressure-area relation: a noninvasively accessible index of regional myocardial contractility. *J Am Coll Cardiol* 1993;21:298A (Abstract).

10. Gorcsan J, 3rd, Romand JA, Mandarino WA, Deneault LG, Pinsky MR: Assessment of left ventricular performance by on-line pressure-area relations using echocardiographic automated border detection. *J Am Coll Cardiol* 1994;23:242-252.

11. Bednarz JE, Marcus RH, Lang RM: Technical guidelines for performing automated border detection studies. *J Am Soc Echocardiogr* 1995;8:293-305.

12. Jarrett JR, Flowers NC: Signal-averaged electrocardiography: history, techniques, and clinical applications. *Clin Cardiol* 1991;14:984-994.

13. Mor-Avi V, Gillesberg IE, Korcarz C, Sandelski J, Lang RM: Improved quantification of left ventricular function by applying signal averaging to echocardiographic acoustic quantification. *J Am Soc Echocardiogr* 1995;8:679-689.

14. Lang RM, Briller RA, Neumann A, Borow KM: Assessment of global and regional left ventricular mechanics: applications to myocardial ischemia. In: Kerber RE, ed: *Echocardiography in Coronary Artery Disease.* Mount Kisco, NY: Futura Publishing Co.; 1988: 1-347.

15. Borow KM, Marcus RH, Neumann A, Lang RM: Modern noninvasive techniques for the assessment of left ventricular systolic performance. In Braunwald E, ed. *Heart Disease: A textbook of Cardiovascular Medicine.* Philadelphia, PA: W. B. Saunders; 1992:31-40.

16. Pombo JF, Troy BL, Tussell RO: Left ventricular volumes and ejection fraction by echocardiography. *Circulation* 1971;43:480-490.

17. Spirito P, Maron BJ, Bonow RO: Noninvasive assessment of left ventricular diastolic function: comparative analysis of Doppler echocardiographic and radionuclide angiographic techniques. *J Am Col Cardiol* 1986;7:518-526.

18. Slutsky RA, Mancini GB, Gerber KH, Carey PH, Ashburn WL, Higgins CB: Radionuclide analysis of ejction time, peak ejection rate, and time to peak ejection rate: response to supine bicycle exercise in normal subjects and in patients with coronary heart disease. *Am Heart J* 1983;105:802-810.

19. Aroney CN, Ruddy TD, Dighero H, Fifer MA, Boucher CA, Palacios IF: Differentiation of restrictive cardiomyopathy from pericardial constriction: assessment of diastolic function by radionuclide angiography. *J Am Coll Cardiol* 1989;13:1007-1014.

20. Bonow RO, Bacharach SL, Green MV, Kent KM, Rosing DR, Lipson LC, Leon MB, Epstein SE. Impaired left ventricular diastolic filling in patients with coronary

artery disease: assessment with radionuclide angiography. *Circulation* 1981;64:315-323.

21. Mancini GB, Slutsky RA, Norris SL, Bhargava V, Ashburn WL, Higgins CB: Radionuclide analysis of peak filling rate, filling fraction, and time to peak filling rate: response to supine bicycle exercise in normal subjects and patients with coronary disease. *Am J Cardiol* 1983;51:43-51.

22. Poliner LR, Farber SH, Glaeser DH, Nylaan L, Verani MS, Robert R: Alteration of diastolic filling rate during exercise radionuclide angiography: a highly sensitive technique for detection of coronary artery disease. *Circulation* 1984;70:942-950.

23. Udelson JE, Bonow RO: Radionuclide angiographic evaluation of left ventricular diastolic function. In Gaasch WH, LeWinter MM, eds. *Left ventricular diastolic dysfunction and heart failure.* Philadelphia, PA: Lea & Febiger; 1994:181-186 .

24. Barbier A, Alioto G, Guazzi M: Left atrial function and ventricular filling in hypertensive patients with paroxysmal atrial fibrillation. *J Am Coll Cardiol* 1994;24:165-170.

25. Triposkiadis F, Tentolouris K, Androulakis A, Trikas A, Toutouzas K, Dyriakidis M, Gialafos J, Toutouzas P: Left atrial mechanical function in the healthy elderly: new insights from a combined assessment of changes in atrial volume and transmitral flow velocity. *J Am Soc Echocardiogr* 1995;8:801-809.

26. Waggoner AD, Barzilai B, Miller JG, Perez J: On-line assessment of left atrial area and function by echocardiographic automatic boundary detection. *Circulation* 1993;88:1142-1149.

27. Coene AJ, Mor-Avi V, Gillesberg IE, Korcarz C, Sandelski J, Lang RM: Noninvasive assessment of left ventricular function in dilated cardiomyopathy using signal averaged echocardiographic acoustic quantification. *J Am Soc Echocardiogr* 1995;8:348 (Abstract).

28. Mor-Avi V, Weinert L, Vignon P, Spencer KT, Lang RM: Assessment of LV function using signal averaged acoustic quantification waveforms under inotropic interventions. *J Am Soc of Echocardiogr* 1996;3:400 (Abstract).

29. Vignon P, Mor-Avi V, Young C, Gillesberg I, Karp R, Aronson S, Lang RM: Intraoperative transesophageal monitoring of LV function using signal averaged acoustic quantification waveforms. *Circulation* 1995;92: I-734 (Abstract).

5 Evaluation of Left Ventricular Diastolic Function Using Acoustic Quantification

Sandra C. Gan and Richard L. Popp

The concept that heart failure and significant cardiac impairment could be attributed to diastolic dysfunction was first introduced by Dougherty *et al.* [1] in 1984. In his study of 188 patients with heart failure, 36% of the patients had normal or near normal left ventricular (LV) systolic function, with ejection fractions of 0.45 or greater. Echocardiographic findings in these patients demonstrated an abnormally low left atrial emptying index which suggested poor left ventricular compliance. As a result, heart failure in these patients was attributed to diastolic dysfunction. Subsequently, Soufer *et al.* [2] confirmed these findings. They reported that 42% of their heart failure patients had intact left ventricular systolic function. Using echocardiographic and radionuclide techniques to assess cardiac function they reported a high incidence of diastolic dysfunction in patients with heart failure symptoms and preserved systolic function.

Although these studies demonstrated that the syndrome of heart failure could be attributed to diastolic dysfunction, identification and quantification of diastolic dysfunction was difficult because effective techniques were not available. This difficulty partially is a consequence of the complicated dynamic phases of diastole. The transition from contraction to relaxation occurs progressively throughout left ventricular ejection. When the heart rate is less than 120 beats per minute and there is sinus rhythm, three phases are described during diastole. The left ventricle fills rapidly during early diastole as a result of a small initial positive diastolic pressure gradient between the left atrium and ventricle, coupled with ventricular relaxation, elastic recoil and/or by inertial properties of the myocardium (or diastolic suction). As the atrium empties and the ventricle fills, the atrioventricular pressure gradient reverses, virtually stopping filling and causing a period of diastasis. Passive slow filling occurs dependent on the compliance of the LV myocardium. In the last phase of diastole, atrial contraction results in a small late diastolic pressure change and further LV filling. Because LV myocardial relaxation continues after mitral valve opening, when blood flows into the left ventricle during rapid filling, any measurements of pressure or volume will reflex the complex interaction between the viscoelastic forces of the myocardium, elastic recoil, as well as the passive compliance of the ventricle.

For practical purposes, measurements of LV diastolic function have been made usually beginning at the time of aortic valve closure. These have included the duration of the isovolumic relaxation period and the rapid filling phase, and have extended to the time of mitral valve closure. Therefore, measurements of myocardial diastolic function have incorporated data extending from the isovolumic relaxation period. Mathematical extrapolation of this phase normally has been done to reflect continued myocardial relaxation after mitral valve opening.

Diastolic Function as Evaluated by Conventional Methods: Ventriculography, Nuclear Medicine, And Doppler

Many investigators have applied left ventriculography, radionuclide studies, and Doppler echocardiography to evaluate left ventricular diastolic function [3-8]. With the use of left ventriculography simultaneous pressures, volumes, and geometry can be measured throughout the cardiac cycle to assess the rate and timing of filling of the ventricle. One can observe the phenomenon known as "checking," which is a visible abrupt cessation in the filling at the time of left ventriculography associated with some types of ventricular diastolic dysfunction. The presence of "checking" is neither a sensitive nor an easily quantifiable marker for diastolic dysfunction. Furthermore, frame by frame analysis of ventriculographic data is cumbersome.

Using nuclear technology, the counts emitted from the left ventricular blood pool are measured over several gated cycles. The rate of increase of counts (or peak filling rate (PFR)) or volume expansion is considered representative of both LV filling and of the rate of relaxation. Measurements of impaired ventricular relaxation by radionuclide techniques include reduced peak filling rate, prolonged time from end systole-to-peak filling rate and increase in the contribution of atrial systole to left ventricular filling [6, 7]. However, these are not always reliable. Diastolic dysfunction could be simulated in normal individuals merely by a change in posture or medication. Plotnick *et al.* [9] demonstrated that measurements of diastolic function may be substantially altered in normal subjects simply by changing from the supine to the upright position. Significant increases in left ventricular peak filling rates have followed the intravenous administration of verapamil compared with baseline measurements in these normal subjects. Thus, these parameters may not be ideal for serial evaluation of diastolic function.

In 1988, Appleton *et al.* [10] studied diastolic function by applying Doppler evaluation of mitral inflow parameters to reflect the blood flow into the left ventricle during diastole. Three abnormal filling patterns were described as assessed by Doppler echocardiography. These include reduced E-wave velocity (initial diastolic filling), decreased mitral flow velocity deceleration time, and increased A wave velocity (atrial contribution). These non invasive indices of diastolic function, like the hemodynamically derived indices, depend not only upon the complex interaction between active and passive properties of the ventricle, but are also greatly affected by loading conditions, heart rate, systolic ventricular function and age [10-13].

Doppler signals of mitral inflow obtained from the mitral valve leaflet tips can be employed to estimate the isovolumic relaxation time (IVRT) and the mitral pressure half-time (PHT) which are measures of diastolic function. The rate of decrease of velocity after the E point has been measured and expressed as the time taken for the initial pressure gradient to fall to one-half of it value (Pressure half-time, PHT), calculated from the modified Bernoulli equation. In the early stages of LV relaxation abnormality the Doppler signals of mitral inflow demonstrate reduction in the amplitude of the early diastolic (E) wave, as well as prolonged deceleration. The A wave is augmented with strong contraction. In more advanced stages of diastolic dysfunction, diastolic filling demonstrates a tall sharp E wave with a brief deceleration time and a small A wave. (Figure 5.1). This method of measuring left ventricular diastolic function has several limitations which are primarily related to dependence of the parameters on loading conditions. Compensatory mechanisms, such as elevated left atrial pressure, may result in the mitral inflow Doppler velocity recordings appearing normal in the presence of diastolic dysfunction (*i.e.* "pseudonormalized") [10]. Therefore, the search for other techniques to quantify left ventricular diastolic function has led several groups to evaluate acoustic quantification (AQ) for this purpose as conventional echocardiographic and Doppler-derived techniques are limited for measurement of diastolic dysfunction.

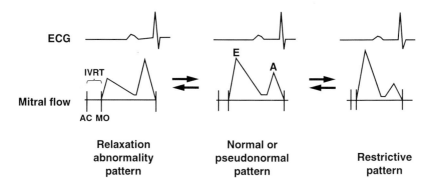

Figure 5.1. Schematic diagram of the spectrum of Doppler mitral flow velocity patterns discussed. The middle panel shows predominance of the early diastolic velocity peak (E-wave) and less prominent velocity during atrial filling (A-wave). Impaired left ventricular relaxation, without compensation, typically shows a pattern of lower E-wave velocity, reduced deceleration slope after the E-wave and a prolonged isovolumic relaxation time (IVRT) (left panel). A "restrictive" filling pattern (right panel) is characterized by an increased E-wave velocity, rapid deceleration slope after the E-wave, a diminutive A-wave and a short isovolumic relaxation time. Abbreviations: AC - aortic valves closure, MO - mitral valve opening, ECG - electrocardiogram. (Redrawn after Appleton, *et al.*, *J Am Coll Cardiol* 1988;12:426-440).

AQ Validated by Doppler-Acquired Parameters

Two-dimensional echocardiographic evaluation of left ventricular size and function has generally remained qualitative and subjective, until recently because computer-assisted systems which are necessary for off-line digital acquisition of selected frames, require tedious and time-consuming manual frame by frame analysis. Acoustic quantification (AQ) uses integrated ultrasonic backscatter processing to automatically detect and delineate the blood-tissue interface and to provide on-line quantitative display of border tracking between endocardium and blood (see Chapter 1). There is also simultaneous display of waveforms quantifying LV area and changes in LV area with respect to time. This relatively new approach calculates and displays fractional blood pool area change and the rate of cavity area change throughout the cardiac cycle in real time [14-16]. With simultaneous display of the waveforms and the two-dimensional images from which the waveforms were obtained, one can visually confirm the accuracy of the border detection which is used to produce the waveform (see Chapter 2). When applied to the left ventricle, the waveform of the AQ area during the cardiac cycle resembles a left ventricular volume curve [18].

Previous studies have validated the accuracy and precision of the software for area measurements both by comparison with manual tracing and by demonstrating reproducibility of these measurements [15,16] (see Chapter 3). Other studies have validated the accuracy of this technique by comparison of measurements of the AQ waveform with established indices of systolic and diastolic ventricular performance [17-23]. Furthermore, pressure-area loops using acoustic quantification-derived areas have been shown to be quantitatively similar to the predicted response of pressure-volume relations to inotropic modulation [24,25] (see Chapter 9). Significant correlations were found between the timing of some phases of the cardiac cycle determined from automated boundary detection of the left ventricle and from Doppler-derived parameters of flow using a transthoracic imaging approach [17-23].

Thus far the major emphasis in on-line AQ of the left ventricle has been the establishment of methods for measuring systolic functional parameters on the basis of alterations in the shape and magnitude of the waveform. Our own studies [17] have demonstrated the correlation of the AQ waveform with the Doppler signal. Thirty-five subjects (between the ages of 30 and 38 years old) were evaluated, of which 16 were healthy volunteers, and the rest having been referred for echocardiographic examination because of mitral valve prolapse (n=4), left ventricular functional assessment (n=4), murmur assessment (n=3), assessment after radiofrequency ablation of accessory conduction tissue bundles (n=3), coronary artery disease (n=2), prior stroke (n=1), suspected cardiomyopathy (n=1) and suspected left ventricular hypertrophy (n=1).

In this study, the following waveform points were used on the AQ curve (Figure 5.2): the point after the atrial contraction (the maximal area) or end diastolic cavity area (EDA) was labeled as point A. The point of end-systolic cavity area (ESA) or minimal cavity area was labeled point C. The onset of early ventricular filling was designated as point D and the end of rapid ventricular filling period was labeled point E. The point at the onset of atrial contraction was designated as point F. All blood pool cavity areas in the AQ data were expressed in cm² and the change in blood pool cavity area per unit time, or dA/dt was expressed in units of cm²/s.

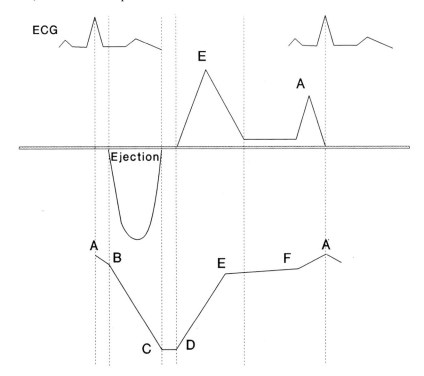

Figure 5.2. Schematic drawing of the time correspondence for diastolic events between the Doppler trace (middle trace) and the waveform from acoustic quantification (lower trace). Electrocardiogram (ECG) is the upper trace. The rapid filling time by Doppler is consistently longer than by the waveform from acoustic quantification. See Figure 5.1 for explanation of abbreviations on the upper trace and see text for explanation of points on the lower trace. (By permission of Chenzbraun et al, *Br Heart J* 1993;70:448-456).

The decrease in cross sectional area of the left ventricle from end diastole to end systole was defined as fractional area change (FAC) and calculated as:

$$FAC = (A \text{ area} - C \text{ area})/A \text{ area}$$

The portion of the total area change that occurred by the end of the rapid filling period was defined as rapid filling fractional area change (RFFAC) and was calculated as:

$$RFFAC = (E \text{ area} - C \text{ area})/(A \text{ area} - C \text{ area})$$

The portion of the total blood pool cavity area change that occurred during atrial contraction was defined as atrial filling fractional area change (AFFAC) and was calculated as:

$$AFFAC = (A \text{ area} - F \text{ area})/(A \text{ area} - C \text{ area})$$

These data (Figure 5.3) were compared to that derived from the early and late filling Doppler flow velocity signals obtained from transmitral flow in normal subjects and from patients.

The "A" wave of the Doppler signal from the mitral valve leaflets corresponded to the smaller increase in blood pool cavity area over time, which is above and beyond the area from early passive LV filling. The systolic and diastolic cavity area values obtained by AQ in normal subjects were measured and correlations of early and atrial filling parameters with AQ waveform and Doppler indices were reported [17]. Abnormal subjects compared to normals demonstrated a more prominent atrial component of the total area change (40% vs 20%) and a slower rate of rapid filling (23 cm²/s vs 35 cm²/s). The patients with abnormal AQ diastolic waveform tracings generally had abnormal relaxation by Doppler criteria.

Intra-observer reproducibility was quite good when assessed for measurements of end diastolic areas (r=0.99, standard error=4%), end systolic areas (r=0.99, standard error = 9%), and rapid filling fractional area change (r=0.83, standard error = 6%). Ten randomly selected, previously videotaped studies were also assessed by a second investigator to obtain inter-observer reproducibility of the same measurements. Good reproducibility was found for all measurements: end diastolic areas (r=0.98, standard error = 3%), end systolic areas areas (r=0.98, standard error = 4%), and rapid filling fractional area change (r=0.72, standard error = 7%).

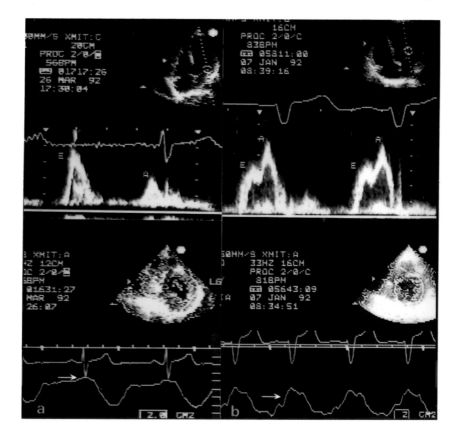

Figure 5.3. Morphology of the waveform from acoustic quantification. Left panels (a) subject with a normal Doppler pattern, right panels (b) patient with an abnormal relaxation pattern. Upper panels: Doppler trace, lower panels, waveforms from acoustic quantification. Arrow: atrial component of ventricular filling. In patient (b) the diastolic filling shows a prominent atrial component, which is of higher amplitude and with a more abrupt upslope that the trace of the normal subject (a) whose filling is represented primarily by the early rapid filling segment. Abbreviations as in Figure 5.1. (By permission from Chenzbraun et al, *Br Heart J* 1993;70:448-456).

Similar findings were confirmed by Foley *et al.* [27] when they compared AQ and Doppler diastolic measurements in 20 individuals (10 normal, 7 with systemic amyloidosis, 2 with Friedrich's ataxia and one with hypertensive left ventricular hypertrophy).

Physiologic Changes in AQ Diastolic Parameters with Aging

There is evidence that elderly subjects also may exhibit alterations in ventricular diastolic function in the absence of overt cardiac disease and as part of the normal aging process [28,29]. In addition to changes in the contractile properties of the aging cardiac muscle, considerable evidence from studies of isolated hearts and myocardium from aging animals suggests there are functionally significant alterations in the compliance and stiffness of the aging heart [20,31]. These changes are probably due to alteration in myocardial collagen [32]. Furthermore, the contractile proteins themselves may develop an increased resistance to separation.

Several studies using Doppler echocardiography [11,13,33,34] demonstrated that the ratio of peak flow velocity during the atrial contraction phase (A wave) to that during the rapid filling phase (E wave) increases significantly with age. The portion of LV filling that occurs during atrial contraction in healthy subjects increases from 12% in a 20 year old man to 46% in an 80 year old woman [34]. Correlation of changes in diastolic ventricular function with aging has also been assessed by observing filling dynamics of pulmonary vein flow into the left atrium and LV inflow velocities [35].

We have acquired baseline AQ data for early and late diastolic filling parameters in healthy subjects over a broad age range as a basis for future comparison with patterns found in cardiac disease. Of 82 volunteers sixteen were excluded because of murmurs (n=2), left bundle branch block (n=2), abnormal two-dimensional or Doppler echocardiogram (n=4) or technically difficult AQ study (n=8). The remaining 66 individuals were considered healthy by history, physical examination, ECG, and two-dimensional and Doppler echocardiography. The following variables were examined: resting heart rate, standard Doppler measurements of isovolumic relaxation time and pressure half-time [10]. Also, AQ parameters of end-systolic LV cavity area (ESA), the rapid filling fractional area change (RFFAC), the atrial filling fractional area change (AFFAC), the mean rate of early rapid filling and duration of early rapid filling. RFFAC is the change in left ventricular area assuring the early rapid filling period of the LV as a fraction of the total area change during that cardiac cycle. AFFAC is the change in LV area which is due to atrial contraction as a fraction of the total area change during that cardiac cycle. The mean, standard deviation and correlation coefficient with standard error of each AQ variable with age were calculated.

In the parasternal short axis view RFFAC declined with increasing age from the third to the ninth decade (from 0.77±0.01 to 0.63±0.04, p=0.0001). In the apical 4-chamber view RFFAC declined with increasing age from the third to the ninth decade (from 0.80±0.05 to 0.63±0.04, p=0.001) (Figure 5.4). The AFFAC increased with increasing age in a complementary fashion (Figure 5.5). The diastolic function values for the healthy subjects reported by Chenzbraun *et al.* [26], show data similar to the values measured in the younger population of our preliminary study described. While both studies were performed at our laboratory, there was no duplication of patients enrolled in either study.

Intra-observer variability demonstrated good reproducibility obtained for measurements of AFFAC in the parasternal short axis and 4 chamber views (r=0.97, standard error = 3% and r=0.98, standard error = 4%, respectively). Twenty randomly selected, previously videotaped studies were also assessed by a second investigator to obtain inter-observer reproducibility of the same measurements. Good reproducibility was found for all the measurements: for measurements of AFFAC in the parasternal short axis and 4 chamber views, inter-observer reproducibility was (r=0.97, standard error = 3%) and (r=0.95, standard error = 5%), respectively.

Since the effect of preload on these measurements was not assessed [12,36], it is not known whether this method is superior to Doppler echocardiography in this context. Of note, we specifically chose to measure age-related ranges for values for LV cavity area instead of LV volume because many of the assumptions regarding LV cavity contour, which are used to derive volume from area measurements, may lead to somewhat inaccurate determination of volumes. The LV volume of hearts of various shapes will have a variable relation to an LV area at a given cross-sectional level.

These data provide an age specific reference for these ventricular filling functional parameters. The results are consistent with other studies which demonstrate that LV distensibility in early diastole is impaired with aging and that there is a compensatory increase in the contribution of the atrial contraction to LV filling. The changes in left ventricular diastolic function associated with aging may become hemodynamically significant as they result in a trend toward dependence of left ventricular filling on atrial contraction. The effects of age on left ventricular diastolic filling as observed in these results suggests that future investigations utilizing AQ to assess left ventricular diastolic function may require the use of age-matched controls subjects.

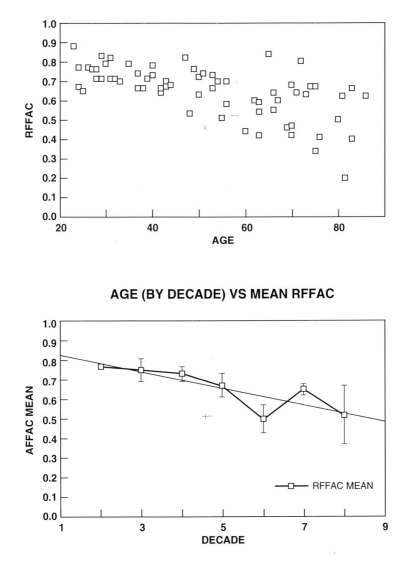

Figure 5.4. Left ventricular rapid filling fractional area change (RFFAC), by acoustic quantification in the apical four-chamber view, plotted versus age from the third to the ninth decade in subjects without recognizable heart disease. Upper panel: values, lower panel: mean values for each decade.

AGE VS AFFAC

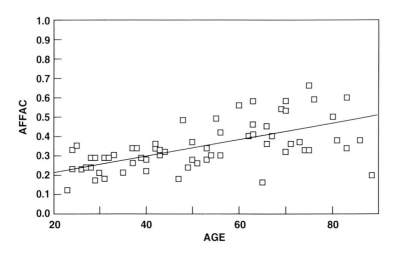

AGE (BY DECADE) VS AFFAC MEAN WITH SD

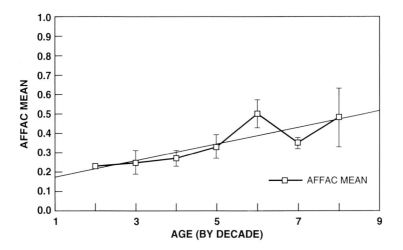

Figure 5.5. Left ventricular atrial filling fractional area change (AFFAC), by acoustic quantification in the apical four-chamber view, plotted versus age from the third to the ninth decade in subjects without recognizable heart disease. Upper panel: values; lower panel: mean values for each decade.

AQ to Recognize Pseudonormalized Doppler Signals

Chenzbraun et al, demonstrated AQ to be a useful tool in identifying Doppler LV filling patterns in patients with LV hypertrophy, particularly in those presumed to have pseudonormalized Doppler mitral inflow signals [26]. In a group of sixteen patients with LV hypertrophy (LVH) (8 with hypertrophic cardiomyopathy, 4 with aortic stenosis and 4 with arterial hypertension), patients were categorized by both the pattern of the transmittal Doppler signal and the AQ tracing of ventricular cavity area. Normal controls demonstrated a Doppler signal with normal E wave, A wave and AQ waveform with large RFFAC and small AFFAC (Figure 5.3,A). Five patients had easily demonstrated diastolic dysfunction using both Doppler mitral inflow signals (E/A<1) and AQ tracings, with a small RFFAC and large AFFAC (Figure 5.3,B). Although there was concordance between Doppler tracings and AQ in the majority of patients; the data were disparate in some of the patients (Figure 5.6). These latter patients presumably had pseudonormalization of their Doppler signals, as the AQ tracings continued to demonstrate an abnormal increase in filling during atrial contraction (Figure 5.7). These data suggest AQ may be complementary to Doppler techniques in the evaluation of diastolic dysfunction.

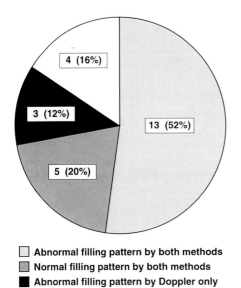

Figure 5.6. Distribution of concordance and discordance of abnormal filling patterns by Doppler echocardiography and acoustic quantification. (By permission of Chenzbraun *et al., J Am Coll Cardiol* 1994;23:1179-1185).

☐ Abnormal filling pattern by both methods
▨ Normal filling pattern by both methods
■ Abnormal filling pattern by Doppler only
☐ Abnormal filling pattern by AQ only

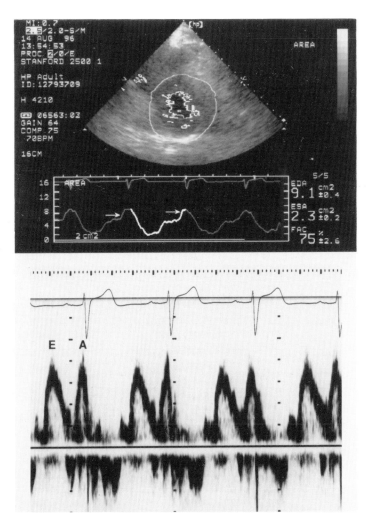

Figure 5.7. Upper panel: Two-dimensional echocardiogram, in the parasternal short axis view, with demarcation of the LV cavity area tracked by AQ (gray wedge, above), and the area waveform below. The tracing is from a patient with mitral regurgitation, LV hypertrophy and suspected LV dysfunction. The diastolic filling by AQ shows a prominent atrial component (arrows) and atrial filling fractional area change that is abnormally large for this patient's age. Lower panel: Mitral inflow Doppler profiles obtained in the same patient show a normalized pattern with E-wave and A-wave of equal amplitude. Abbreviations: EDA - end diastolic area, ESA - end systolic area, FAC - fractional area change.

Potential Pitfalls in Using AQ

There are potential pitfalls which might influence the AQ derived waveforms when applying AQ for the purpose of obtaining pressure-area loops [24,25]. There is "a 1±1 frame delay", (*i.e.* a 0 to 2 frame delay), as images are obtained and placed into a buffer while AQ calculations are made for displaying the waveforms on the screen as per manufacturer. Experiments by Keren *et al.*, have shown that the AQ delay relative to high fidelity pressure recordings ranges from 20 to 34 ms and 35 to 57 ms at echocardiographic frame rates of 60/sec and 33/sec, respectively [37]. Therefore, depending on the echocardiographic image frame rate, there may be a 33 to 66 ms delay between the two-dimensional image and AQ waveform. This delay was not significantly influenced by the type of transducer used, distance from the region of interest or size of the region of interest. The delay in the AQ signal relative to the echocardiographic image, ranges from nil to less than one frame duration, whereas it is delayed one to two frame durations relative to the electrocardiogram as processed by the imaging system. Attempts to use electrocautery to assist timing were unsuccessful as there is no time delay between electrocautery use and signal transmission to the AQ screen; the signal from electrocautery is transmitted instantaneously through the recording equipment.

Sonomicrometers which are commonly utilized in experimental animal settings to measure cardiac chamber dimension were found to introduce both ultrasonic and electronic noise which interfered with the ultrasound signal used to create the AQ waveforms information. These studies suggested that modifications in the equipment used could overcome this difficulty [37].

Studies of left heart dynamics in experimental animals is facilitated by the use of a right heart bypass pump in order to control the preload and afterload of the left heart. However, Keren, et. al., found use of such a device introduced a large number of ultrasonic targets within the chambers of interest. Presumably these targets represented microbubbles and/or particles within the blood cavity that result from its passage through the bypass pump. Similar difficulties were encountered in the *in vitro* experiments using a pump connected to a balloon as an approach to simulate a cardiac chamber. While there may be ways to decrease such spontaneous echo contrast from the use of these pumps, the investigators found it easiest to avoid this experimental design and to study the physiologic parameters of interest by other means [37].

Another concern raised by this study was that during the creation of pressure-area loops the relatively "noisy" digitized AQ signal has to be considerably smoothed and averaged. Therefore no fine incisural points were seen, thus potentially obscuring small rapid changes in cavity area. This investigation did not specifically study the recognition of discrete events within the cardiac cycle by means of the AQ tracing displayed with the pressure tracing, however, such noise remains a potential limitation of the method.

Future Applications of AQ

In early work reported so far, AQ seems a reliable, cost-effective and time efficient method that can provide quantitative serial evaluation of the dynamics of ventricular diastole. Although there are limitations to this technique, many of these factors can be minimized through operator experience. With the expanding use of cardiac ultrasound by cardiologists, anesthesiologists and surgeons, investigation of this new approach may allow reliable comparison of quantitative data related to ventricular diastolic function. The use of AQ should not only improve our understanding of cardiac physiology and pathophysiology, but should also be useful in the guidance and assessment of therapy to treat and correct diastolic dysfunction.

References

1. Dougherty AH, Naccarelli GV, Gray EL, Hicks CH and Goldstein RA: Congestive heart failure with normal systolic function. *Am J Cardiol* 1984;54:778-782.
2. Soufer R, Wohlgelernter D, Vita NA, Amuchestegui M, Sostman HD, Berger HJ, Zarel BL: Intact systolic left ventricular function in clinical congestive heart failure. *Circulation* 1985;55:1032-1036.
3   Lew W: Evaluation of left ventricular diastolic function. *Circulation* 1989;79:1393-1397.
4. Bianco JA, Filiberti AW, Baker SP, King MA, Nalwaika LA, Leahey D, Doherty PW, Alpert JS: Ejection fraction and heart rate correlate with diastolic peak filling rate at rest and during exercise. *Chest* 1985;88:107-113.
5. Bianco JA, Bachrach SL, Greene MV: Impaired left ventricular diastolic filling in patient with coronary artery disease: Assessment with radionuclide angiography. *Circulation* 1981;64:315-323.
6. Bonow RO: Noninvasive evaluation of left ventricular diastolic function by radionuclide angiography: limitations and application. *Int J Cardiol* 1984;5:659-663.
7. Iskandrian AS, Heo J, Segal BL, Askenase A: Left ventricular diastolic function: evaluation by radionuclide angiography. *Am Heart J* 1988;115:924-929.
8. Spirito P, Maron BJ, Bonow RO: Noninvasive assessment of left ventricular

diastolic function: comparative analysis of Doppler echocardiographic and radionuclide techniques. *J Am Coll Cardiol* 1986;7:518-526.

9. Plotnick GD, Kahn B, Rogers WJ, Fisher ML, Becker LC: Effect of postural changes, nitroglycerin and verapamil on diastolic function as determined by radionuclide angiography in normal subjects. *J Am Coll Cardiol* 1988;12:121-129.

10. Appleton CP, Hatle LK, Popp RL: Relation of transmittal flow velocity patterns to left ventricular diastolic function: new insights from a combined hemodynamic and Doppler echocardiographic study. *J Am Coll Cardiol* 1988;12:426-440.

11. Miyatake K, Okamoto M, Kinoshita N, Owa M, Nakasone I, Sakakibara H, Nimura Y: Augmentation of atrial contribution to left ventricular inflow with aging as assessed by intracardiac Doppler flowmetry. *Am J Cardiol* 1984;53:586-589.

12. Choong CY, Hermann HC, Weyman AE, Fifer MA: Preload dependence of Doppler-derived indexes of left ventricular diastolic function in humans. *J Am Coll Cardiol* 1987;10:800-808.

13. Gardin JM, Rohan MK, Davidson DM, Dabestani A, Sklansky M, Garcia R, Knoll ML, White DB, Gardin SK: Doppler transmittal flow velocity parameters; relationship between age, body surface area, blood pressure and gender in normal subjects. *Am J Noninvasive Cardiol* 1987;1:3-10.

14. Pérez JE, Waggoner AD, Barzilai B, Melton HE, Miller JG, Sobel BE: On-line assessment of ventricular function by automatic boundary detection and ultrasonic backscatter imaging. *J Am Coll Cardiol* 1992;19:313-320.

15. Pérez JE, Klein SC, Prater DM, Fraser CE, Cardona H, Waggoner AD, Holland MR, Miller JG, Sobel BE: Automated, on-line quantification of left ventricular dimensions and function by echocardiography with backscatter imaging and lateral gain compensation. *Am J Cadiol* 1992;70:1200-1205.

16. Vandenberg BF, Rath LS, Stuhlmuller P, Melton HE, Skorton DJ: Estimation of left ventricular cavity area with an on-line, semiautomated echocardiographic edge detection system. *Circulation* 1992;86:159-166.

17. Chenzbraun A, Pinto FJ, Milton S, Schnittger I, Popp RL: Noninvasive assessment of left ventricular diastolic function by acoustic quantification. *Br Heart J* 1993;70:448-456.

18. Gorcsan J III, Mortia S, Mandarino WA: Two dimensional echocardiography automated border detection accurately reflects changes in left ventricular volume. *J Am Soc Echocardiogr* 1993;6:482-489.

19. Gorcsan J III, Lazar JR, Romand J, Pinsky MR: On-line estimation of stroke volume using echocardiographic automated border detection in the canine left ventricle. *Am Heart J* 1993;125:1316-1323.

20. Stewart WJ, Rodkey SM, Gunawardena S: Left ventricular volume calculation with integrated backscatter from echocardiography. *J Am Soc Echocardiogr* 1993;6:553-563.

21. Morrissey RL, Siu SC, Guerreo JL, Newell JB, Weyman AE, Picard MH: Automated assessment of ventricular volume and function by echcoadiography: Validation of automated border detection. *J Am Soc Echocardiogr* 1994;7:107-115.

22. Stoddard MF, Keedy DL, Longaker RA: Two-dimensional transesophageal echo-

87885

quantification: Comparison with pulsed Doppler echocardiography. *J Am Soc
Echocardiogr* 1994;7:116-131.

23. Gottlieb S, Keren A, Khoury Z, Stern S: Findings of automatic border detection in
    subjects with left ventricular diastolic dysfunction by Doppler echocardiography. *J
    Am Soc Echocardiogr* 1995;8:149-161.
24. Gorcsan J III, Romand JA, Mandarino WA, Deneault LG, Pinsky MR: Assessment
    of left ventricular performance by on-line pressure-area relations using
    echocardiographic automated border detection. *J Am Coll Cardiol* 1994;23:242-252.
25. Gorcsan J III, Gasior TA, Mandarino WA, Deneault LG, Hattler BG, Pinsky MR:
    Assessment of the immediate effects of cardiopulmonary bypass on left ventricular
    performance by on-line pressure-area relations. Circulation 1994;89:189-190.
26. Chenzbraun A, Pinto FJ, Popylisen S, Schnittger I, Popp, RL: Filling patterns in left
    ventricular hypertrophy: a combined acoustic quantification and Doppler study. *J
    Am Coll Cardiol* 1994;23:1179-1185.
27. Foley AD, Stewart JB, Tajik AJ: Assessment of left ventricular diastolic function
    with a new automated echocardiographic border detection system: comparison with
    Doppler. *J Am Coll Cardiol* 1992;19:261A (Abstract).
28. Harrison T, Dixon K, Russell R, Bidwai P, Coleman H: The relation of age to the
    duration of contraction, ejection, and relaxation of the normal human heart. *Am
    Heart J* 1964;67:189-199.
29. Dock W: Presbycardia or aging of the myocardium. *NY State J Med* 1945;45:983-
    986.
30. Arora R, Machac J, Goldman M, Butler R, Gorlin R, Horowitz S: Atrial kinetics and
    left ventricular diastolic filling in the healthy elderly. *J Am Coll Cardiol*
    1987;9:1255-1260.
31. Kitzman DW, Edwards WE: Age related changes in the anatomy of the normal
    human heart. *Gerontol Medical Sciences* 1990;45:M33-39.
32. Weber KT: Cardiac interstitium in health and disease: the fibrillar collagen network.
    J Am Coll Cardiol 1989;13:1637-1652.
33. Bryg R, Williams G and Labovitz A: Effect of aging on left ventricular diastolic
    filling in normal subjects. *Am J Cardiol* 1987;59:971-974.
34. Kuo L, Quinones M, Rokey R, Sartori M, Abinader E and Zoghbi W: Quantification
    of atrial contribution to left ventricular filling by Doppler echocardiography and the
    effect of age in normal and diseased hearts. *Am J Cardiol* 1987;59:1174-1178.
35. Klein AL, Burstow DJ, Tajik AJ, Zachariah PK, Bailey KR, Seward JB: Effects of
    age on left ventricular dimensions and filling dynamics in 117 normal persons.
    Mayo Clin Proc 1994;69:212-214.
36. Bahler RC, Margin P: Effects of loading conditions and inotropic state on rapid
    filling phase of left ventricle. *Am J Physiol* 1985;248:H523-H533.
37. Keren A, DeAnda A, Komeda M, Tye T, Handen CR, Daughters GT, Ingels NB,
    Miller C, Popp RL, Nikolic SD: Pitfalls in creation of left atrial pressure-area
    relationships using automated border detection. *J Am Soc Echocardiogr* 1995;8:669-
    678.

aortic pressure (P_{ao}) to flow (Q_{ao}), is a comprehensive characterization of this hydraulic load [20-24]. Z_{in} can be separated into two components: a steady term commonly known as systemic vascular resistance (*SVR*) and a pulsatile component. Since *SVR* is relatively easy to obtain and physically interpretable (i.e., arteriolar properties), it is often the only parameter used in the clinical setting to quantify arterial hydraulic load. The concept of pulsatile load is more difficult to grasp, both in terms of its physical bases and its contribution to aortic pressure–flow relationships. Physically, pulsatile load originates from both geometric (branching topology, bifurcations, geometric taper) and material (wall stiffness and its variation along the arterial tree, elastic taper) properties of the vessels and the fluid contained within (viscosity, inertia). Quantitation of pulsatile arterial load can be made at two levels: global (i.e., properties belonging to the entire circulation downstream from the point of measurement) and regional (i.e., properties belonging to an anatomically well–defined region). Although Z_{in} is the comprehensive characterization of arterial hydraulic load, its relative complexity (i.e., a set of complex numbers in the frequency domain) and the need to acquire instantaneous P_{ao} and Q_{ao} have limited the use of this index in the clinical setting. Consequently, simplified models are often used to calculate reduced number of parameters and to facilitate physiological interpretation of Z_{in}. Global arterial compliance (*AC*) is one such parameter commonly defined in terms of a single lumped quantity, a Windkessel compliance [25-27]. *AC* is generally estimated either from the diastolic aortic pressure decay [27] or by fitting instantaneous pressure and flow data over the entire cardiac cycle [28]. Other characterizations of global pulsatile arterial load include indices of wave reflection (e.g., reflection coefficient spectrum, forward and backward waves) [29]. The regional characterization of pulsatile load includes characteristic impedance (Z_c), pulse wave velocity (*PWV*), and measures of local distensibility and wall stiffness derived from lumen diameter (or area)–pressure relationships. Global characterization is useful when quantifying the hydraulic vascular load imposed on the LV. However, global indices often do not have an identifiable anatomical counterpart and multiple physical processes contribute to a given global index. Therefore, changes in global indices are difficult to interpret in terms of their physical bases. In contrast, regional indices are more suitable for examining the physical properties of the vasculature; although one has to account for their dependence on vascular geometry and distending pressure. Thus, a simultaneous assessment of regional and global indices is needed to understand both the physical bases of pulsatile load and its relevance to the performance of the coupled LV–arterial system in normal and pathological conditions.

Regional Mechanical Properties of the Aorta

Despite the understanding that altered regional mechanical properties of the aortic wall play a role in modifying the optimal interrelationship between aortic pressure, flow, and dimensions and, hence, in determining the coupling between the left ventricle and the systemic circulation in diverse physiologic and disease states, routine evaluation of these properties have been hampered by the technical difficulties encountered in simultaneously acquiring instantaneous aortic pressure, dimension, and wall thickness data [30]. As a consequence, *in vivo* evaluation of regional aortic properties has been limited primarily to animal experiments using methods such as pressure gauges and ultrasonic or electrical dimension gauges for measurements of lumen pressure and external aortic diameter, respectively [31-38]. In humans, aortic elastic properties have been examined using excised vessels or vessel strips [2,32,39]. More recently, diameter–pressure or volume–pressure relationships of the human aorta have been investigated using methodologies such as angiography [17,40,41], impedance catheter [42], and catheter–mounted ultrasonic crystals [43]. Aortic diameter–pressure data acquired over a wide range of loads have been used to differentiate between passive (pressure–dependent) and non–passive (muscle tone and/or structural) determinants of altered elastic properties, both in animal [34,36,44] and human [43] settings. Changes in aortic elastic properties resulting solely from aortic pressure reduction will be evidenced as a shift of the operating point along the baseline diameter–pressure relationship. In contrast, contributions of non–passive mechanisms, such as drug–induced changes of the aortic elastic properties, will be reflected as either rightward or leftward shifts of the aortic diameter–pressure relationship. Pulse wave velocity, measured over a finite length of an arterial segment, has also been used as an index of vessel wall elastic properties [4,6,45,46]. Along with its dependence on vessel geometry and distending pressure, this index provides information on the average stiffness of an arterial segment over which the pulse wave travels. Invasive methods, although technically feasible, preclude serial assessments in the human setting.

Recent technological advances have enabled noninvasive acquisition of vessel dimensional and pressure data required to calculate vessel elastic properties [30,47-51]. The next section describes how measurements of aortic lumen area, derived from transesophageal echocardiographic imaging and automated border detection, can be used with calibrated subclavian pulse tracings and two–dimensionally targeted M–mode measurements of aortic wall thickness to quantify regional mechanical properties of the human aorta.

Methodological Considerations

Determination of Instantaneous Aortic Cross–sectional Area

Instantaneous aortic lumen area measurements can be obtained using the automated border detection system (i.e., Acoustic Quantification) described by Perez *et al.* [52,53], which analyzes the ultrasonic backscatter signal to detect blood/tissue interface in real time (see Chapter 1). We [30,54] and others [50] have applied the identical algorithm previously used to characterize left ventricular performance to transesophageal short–axis views of the descending aorta to obtain instantaneous aortic cross–sectional lumen areas (Figure 6.1). The anatomic proximity between the aorta and the multiplane transesophageal transducer allows acquisition of optimal short–axis views of the proximal

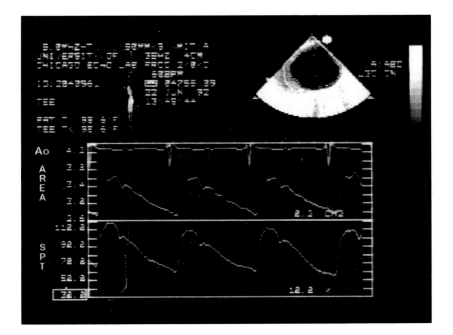

Figure 6.1. Instantaneous aortic cross–sectional area (cm^2, upper tracing labeled Ao AREA) obtained with transesophageal echocardiography with automated border detection (two–dimensional short–axis view) and aortic pressure waveform (mmHg, lower tracing labeled SPT), obtained using a calibrated subclavian pulse tracing. Data are from a human subject.

descending thoracic aorta. To optimize the aortic endothelial border detection it is necessary to properly adjust the overall gain and near field time–gain compensation. Gain adjustments are considered optimal when the tracking line closely follows the real–time endothelial border motions [55]. Because automated border detection processing is based on sampled measurements performed at the end of each acoustic frame, there is a variable time delay between the aortic pressure and area signals. The exact delay is currently difficult to predict with accuracy, but it never exceeds the duration of one echocardiographic frame. We recommend assigning a fixed offset to the pressure waveforms equivalent to 33 milliseconds, corresponding to the duration of one frame when operating at 33 Hz [30,54]. Using this arbitrary offset, the morphology and direction of the area–pressure loops is physiological and similar to that obtained with invasive methodology (*vide infra*). The instantaneous lumen area signal can be digitized on–line via a port option recently incorporated into the ultrasound machine (SONOS 2500, Hewlett Packard) that provides an electrical analog output of the signal.

Determination of Instantaneous Aortic Wall Thickness

Until recently, acquisition of instantaneous aortic wall thickness *in vivo* was technically difficult. This hampered the determination of aortic wall stress required for the computation of incremental elastic modulus, a measure of arterial wall stiffens (*vide infra*). We recently proposed the combined use of (1) transesophageal M–mode measurements of diastolic aortic wall thickness with (2) instantaneous lumen aortic area obtained with the aid of the automated border detection algorithm to calculate instantaneous aortic wall thickness (see Equation 6) [30]. The physical assumptions required for this calculation include incompressibility of the aortic wall and minimal longitudinal aortic deformation during the cardiac cycle, both of which have been shown to be reasonable assumptions [56]. To obtain wall thickness measurements, it is necessary to carefully place the cursor in an area devoid of protruding atherosclerotic plaque. M–mode tracings should be used for measurement only when a continuos line of the posterior wall endothelium is visualized [30,54]. Measurements should be made at the time of the R wave of the ECG (Figure 6.2).

Slama *et al.* [57] recently validated the use of transesophageal echocardiography (5 MHz probe) for measurements of aortic wall thickness. These authors compared thickness obtained by histological measurement with those obtained with transesophageal probe in human aortic specimens and found an excellent agreement between the two methods (r = 0.94; bias = -0.09 mm; precision = 0.19 mm or 11%). Their *in vitro* measurements (1.7± 0.25 mm) are similar to our in vivo measurements (1.7± 0.35 mm).

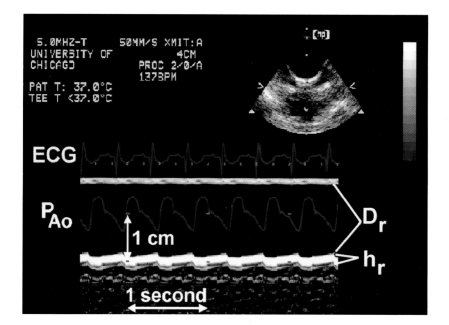

Figure 6.2. Two–dimensionally targeted transesophageal M–mode short–axis view of the canine aorta together with the electrocardiogram (ECG) and invasive, high–fidelity aortic pressure (P_{ao}). D_r and h_r denote aortic diameter and wall thickness, respectively, measured at the time of the R wave of ECG.

Noninvasive Determination of Instantaneous Aortic Pressure

Instantaneous central aortic pressures can be estimated noninvasively from calibrated subclavian or carotid pulse tracings. Previously, we have recorded these pulse tracings using a small plastic funnel positioned over the right subclavian artery at its point of maximal impulse in the supraclavicular fossa and connected by silastic tubing to a strain gauge transducer (model 03040170, Cambridge Instruments) [58]. Pulse tracings can also be recorded with applanation tonometry [59] using a solid–state strain gauge transducer (e.g., SPT–301, Millar Instruments) [60].

We have previously demonstrated that the morphology of the subclavian pulse tracing is similar to that of high–fidelity ascending aortic pressure recordings (Figure 6.3) over a wide range of ages, blood pressures and aortic flows [58]. Similar observations have been made by other investigators [61,62]. Assuming that the electrical output of the strain gauge transducer is linearly proportional to pressure, two points are needed to calibrate the subclavian (or carotid) pulse tracing (i.e., conversion of electrical to physical units). In the past, we equated systolic (P_s) and diastolic (P_d) blood pressures, measured at the brachial artery using an oscillometric sphygmomanometer–based system (e.g., Dinamap Vital Signs monitor, model 1846 SX, Critikon Inc.), to the maximum and minimum, of the pulse tracing respectively. Although the assumption of equal diastolic pressures at central and peripheral locations is reasonable [6,62], systolic pressures can be significantly different due to peripheral pulse wave amplification [63]. Since viscous losses are minimal, it is better to use equality of mean (instead of systolic) pressures at the two location as the second calibration point. Mean brachial artery pressure can be obtained in two ways. One can record the brachial artery pulse tracing (applanation tonometry), calibrate it using the oscillometric systolic and diastolic pressures, and finally,

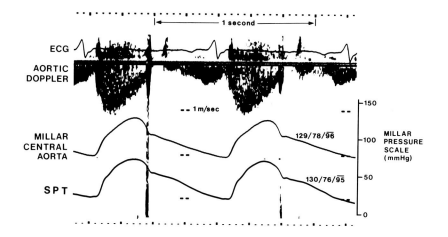

Figure 6.3. Simultaneous pressure tracings acquired noninvasively (calibrated subclavian pulse tracings, SPT) and invasively (Millar catheter–tip micromanometer positioned in the ascending aorta) from a human subject. Note the similarity in the morphology of the two pressure tracings. Also shown are ascending aortic blood velocity (aortic Doppler) and electrocardiogram (ECG).

calculate the mean of this calibrated waveform. Alternatively, the mean can be approximated by using the 2/3–1/3 rule (mean = 2/3 P_d + 1/3 P_s). In summary, the mean and diastolic brachial artery pressures (in physical units) are equated to the mean and minimum of the subclavian (or carotid) pulse tracing (in electrical units), respectively. Instantaneous pressures can then be calculated throughout the cardiac cycle by linear inter– or extrapolation.

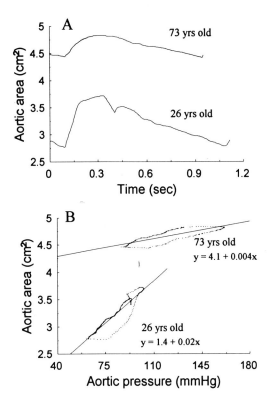

Figure 6.4. Pulsatile changes in aortic area (panel A) and aortic area–pressure loops (panel B) obtained in a 26 year old and a 73 year old patient. Note the increased mean value and reduced pulsatility for aortic area in the elderly subject. The decreased slope of the aortic area–pressure regression obtained from the entire loop denotes lower compliance per unit length in the elderly subject. Modified with permission from the American Heart Association, *Circulation* 1994; 90:1875–1882.

Aortic Area–Pressure Loops

Loop patterns having hysteresis are generated when aortic area and pressure signals are plotted against each other during the entire cardiac cycle (Figure 6.4). The morphologic features of these aortic area–pressure loops, such as the slope of the regression line, width of the hysteresis, and area contained within the loop, provide physiologic insights into the viscoelastic properties of the vessel wall. Similar to previous studies [34,36,42], the aortic area–pressure loops generated with the Acoustic Quantification methodology are elliptical in shape and counterclockwise in direction (Figure 6.4). In contrast to the clockwise direction of the volume–pressure lobp generated by an actively contracting ventricle, the counterclockwise direction of the aortic area–pressure loops denotes the passive behavior of the aorta. The linear regression slope of the entire loop reflects the compliance per unit length estimated over the pressure range of one cardiac cycle (*vide infra*). The width of the hysteresis loop is indicative of vessel wall viscosity and the area contained within the loop corresponds to the energy dissipated locally. We have not performed a quantitative analysis of viscous properties because of the previously described uncertainties regarding the temporal synchronization between the Acoustic Quantification area waveform and pressure signal and relatively low temporal resolution of the two–dimensional imaging (typical frame rate of 30 Hz). In the future, technical enhancements will overcome these current limitations and allow the examination of both elastic and viscous properties from aortic area–pressure loops. In the following sections we will focus on the quantitation of elastic properties only.

Calculation of Aortic Elastic Properties

Aortic dimension (volume, area, or diameter)–transmural pressure relationship contains the information regarding wall elastic properties. Over most of the dimension–pressure range, the greater the change in pressure, the greater the change in aortic dimension. The simplest measure of this physical phenomenon is the aortic volume compliance, C_v (ml/mmHg):

$$C_v = \frac{\Delta V}{\Delta P}, \qquad (1)$$

where, ΔV and ΔP are the change in aortic luminal volume and transmural pressure, respectively. For negligible longitudinal deformation, Equation 1 can be rewritten to express volume compliance per unit length, C_v' (cm^2/mmHg):

$$C_v' = \frac{\Delta A}{\Delta P}, \tag{2}$$

where, ΔA is the change in aortic luminal cross–sectional area. Aortic area (volume)–pressure relationship is typically nonlinear such that volume compliance decreases as the operating pressure increases. However, for small pressure variations around a set–point (e.g., during a cardiac cycle) area (volume)–pressure relationships are reasonably linear and therefore volume compliances can be calculated as the slope of these linear relationships. It should be noted that although arterial compliance (AC) computed from aortic pressure and flow data and C_v have the same units (ml/mmHg), they are not equivalent. As discussed earlier, AC is a global property (belonging to the entire circulation) and C_v is a regional property (belonging to the measurement site). In addition, AC is not simply a sum of volume compliances of all vascular segments; other physical processes (e.g., wave propagation and reflections) are involved in the determination of AC [64].

   Both wall elastic properties and vessel geometry (lumen dimensions and wall thickness) determine volume compliance. Several measures of vascular wall elastic properties, calculated from the measured pressure and dimensional data, are available. For a thick–wall, isotropic elastic tube with uniform diameter and thickness, negligible longitudinal deformation, and incompressible wall (i.e., Poisson's ratio = 0.5), the incremental elastic modulus (E_{inc}, mmHg or dyne/cm^2) for radial deformations at the inner wall is given by [65,66]:

$$E_{inc} = \frac{0.375\,D(D+2h)^2}{h\,(D+h)}\frac{\Delta P}{\Delta D}, \tag{3}$$

where, D and h are the lumen diameter and wall thickness, respectively, and ΔP and ΔD are the changes in lumen pressure and diameter, respectively. Alternatively, Pagani et al. [34] derived the following expression for E_{inc}, computed at the mid–wall:

$$E_{inc} = 0.75 D_m \frac{d\sigma_m}{dD_m}, \qquad (4)$$

where, D_m is the mid–wall diameter ($D_m = D + h$) and mid–wall stress (σ_m) is given by:

$$\sigma_m = 0.5P \left(\frac{D^2(D+2h)^2}{h(D+h)^3} \right). \qquad (5)$$

Both expressions for E_{inc} (Equations 3 and 4) require the measurement of vessel wall thickness. Assuming incompressible aortic wall and negligible longitudinal deformation, aortic muscle area (A_{musc}) remains unchanged throughout the cardiac cycle. By measuring wall thickness at one time–point in the cardiac cycle (e.g., R wave of ECG), one can express instantaneous aortic wall thickness [$h(t)$] in terms of measured instantaneous lumen area [$A(t)$] and A_{musc}.

$$h(t) = \sqrt{\frac{A(t)+A_{musc}}{\pi}} - \sqrt{\frac{A(t)}{\pi}}, \quad A_{musc} = \pi \times h_r \times (D_r + h_r), \quad (6)$$

where, D_r and h_r are the lumen diameter and wall thickness measured at the R wave, respectively. The stress–strain relationship for the aortic wall is typically nonlinear: E_{inc} increases as the vessel is distended. Therefore, intervessel wall stiffness comparisons should be made at matched conditions, e.g., the same level of wall stress.

It is often difficult to measure aortic wall thickness accurately (e.g., when images are obtained using transthoracic echocardiography). Therefore, several indices of wall elastic stiffness have been developed that use lumen pressure and internal dimensions only. Peterson *et al.* [67] proposed one such index, termed the pressure–strain elastic modulus (E_p, mmHg or dyne/cm^2).

$$E_p = \frac{\Delta P}{\frac{\Delta D}{D_d}} = \frac{P_s - P_d}{\frac{D_s}{D_d} - 1} = \frac{P_s - P_d}{\sqrt{\frac{A_s}{A_d}} - 1}, \qquad (7)$$

where, ΔP is the difference between systolic (P_s) and diastolic (P_d) aortic pressures, D_s and D_d and A_s and A_d are systolic (maximum) and diastolic (minimum) lumen diameters and areas, respectively. Another commonly used wall stiffness index (β, dimensionless) was proposed by Hayashi *et al.* [68].

$$\beta \; = \; \frac{ln\left(\dfrac{P_s}{P_d}\right)}{\dfrac{D_s - D_d}{D_{ref}}} \; = \; \frac{ln\left(\dfrac{P_s}{P_d}\right)}{\dfrac{\sqrt{A_s} - \sqrt{A_d}}{\sqrt{A_{ref}}}} , \qquad (8)$$

where, the subscript "*ref*" denotes a reference condition (often taken to be at lumen pressure of 100 mmHg). Approximate values of β can be calculated by replacing D_{ref} by D_d [11,13,69]. Although E_p and β do not require wall thickness measurements, one has to be careful while using them for intervessel comparisons of the elastic properties, especially in situations wherein large variations in vessel radius–to–thickness ratio occur [56].

Validation of the Noninvasive Methodology

Aging and Aortic Elastic Properties

Age–related changes in arterial elastic properties have been well–characterized in previous studies [3-5,7,50]. To validate the noninvasive methodology described earlier, we examined the age–dependency of aortic elastic properties in 25 human subjects undergoing transesophageal echocardiography [30]. In agreement with earlier reports, this study found an inverse relation between C_v' (compliance per unit length) and age (Figure 6.5). C_v' is determined by both the geometry of the vessel (e.g., mid–wall radius, R_m) and stiffness of the wall (e.g., E_{inc}); each of which can be assessed with the noninvasive methodology described above. We examined the age–dependency of R_m and E_{inc} values obtained in individual subjects at a common level of aortic mid–wall stress. R_m increased with age; however, the correlation was weak (r = 0.44). In contrast, E_{inc} was strongly correlated with age (r = 0.78). E_{inc}–age relationship followed a nonlinear function with a marked increase in the steepness after the age of sixty years (Figure 6.5).

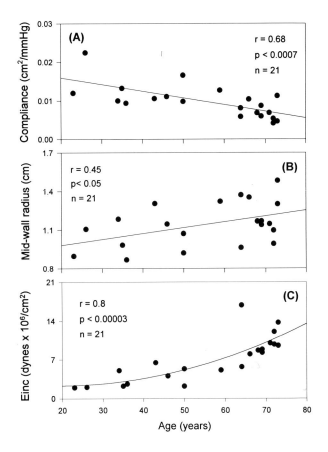

Figure 6.5. Compliance per unit length (panel A), aortic mid–wall radius (panel B) and incremental elastic modulus (E_{inc}) plotted as a function of age. Data are from human subjects and mid–wall radius and E_{inc} values are at a common level of stress stress (0.666×10^{6} dyne/cm^2). Reproduced with permission from the American Heart Association, *Circulation* 1994; 90:1875–1882.

Transesophageal echocardiography–based *in vivo* measurements of aortic external radius (R_o) are similar to previously reported values [70]. However, our *in vivo* values for the h/R_o ratios are higher than those obtained by Learoyd and Taylor [2] *in vitro*, indicating that transesophageal echocardiography–based aortic wall thickness measurements are slightly higher than those obtained *in vitro.* This discrepancy may be related to the inability of echocardiography to discriminate between aortic wall adventitia and the thin layer of perivascular tissue. An alternative explanation may be the occurrence of an artifactual thinning of the vessel wall occurring *in vitro.*

Our *in vivo* E_{inc} values are comparable to the *in vitro* values reported by Learoyd and Taylor [2] on segments of human thoracic aorta. Similarly, the group average for E_p obtained in our study is similar to previously published data [49,51]. However, in a cohort of normotensive patients, Isnard *et al.* [49] failed to observe a correlation between age and aortic arch stiffness (quantified in terms of E_p). The probable explanation for 'this discrepancy is that the patients reported by Isnard *et al.* [49] were all younger than 52 years, a range of age over which E_{inc} appears to remain relatively constant (Figure 6.5).

Regional Variations of Aortic Elastic Properties

We further validated the use of transesophageal echocardiography with automated border detection to quantify vessel elastic properties by measuring regional variations of aortic elastic properties [54]. In nine anesthetized, closed–chest dogs, aortic pressure (catheter–tip transducer, Millar Instruments) and lumen area (transesophageal echocardiography with automated border detection) signals were recorded simultaneously at two aortic sites: just distal to the branching site of the left subclavian artery (proximal) and at the level of the diaphragm (distal). Data were acquired over a range of loading conditions, generated by inferior vena caval balloon occlusion. Aortic area–pressure relationships were found to be linear for both the proximal and distal thoracic aorta (Figure 6.6), indicating that compliance per unit length (C_v') was constant over the range of loading conditions examined. In contrast, other investigators have reported a nonlinear dimension–pressure relationship in dogs, especially at extremely high aortic pressures induced by aortic balloon occlusions [36,44].

C_v' of the proximal aorta was higher than that of the distal descending thoracic aorta (Figure 6.6). Tapering of the distal thoracic aorta was evidenced by a 26% decrease in mid–wall radius between the proximal and distal aortic sites. E_{inc} at common mid–wall stress was greater distally and E_p values for the proximal and distal thoracic aorta compared favorably to those derived by Milnor [56] from invasively acquired pressure-dimension data of Pieper and Paul [71]. These findings are also in agreement with those of Peterson *et al.* [67] and Patel *et al.* [72] who reported a progressive increase in E_p and tapering in diameter along the thoracic aorta. The stiffening of vessel wall can be attributed to the 50% increase in the collagen content of the aortic wall between the arch and diaphragmatic thoracic aorta. Both greater wall stiffness and smaller radius contribute to the lower C_v' values at the distal site.

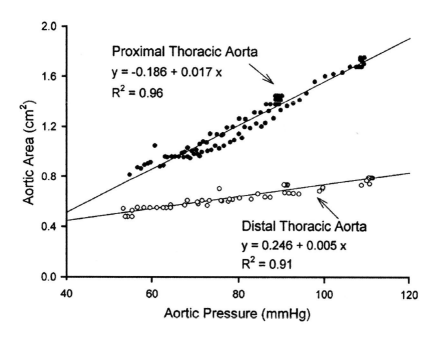

Figure 6.6. Aortic area–pressure relationships at two aortic sites obtained in a dog. Data were collected over a range of pressure values generated by transient inflation of a balloon placed in the inferior vena cava. Reproduced with permission from the American Society of Echocardiography, *J Am Soc Echocardiogr* 1996; 9:539–548.

Physiological Relevance of Aortic Elastic Properties

Convincing evidence exists indicating that aortic elastic properties change in a variety of physiological and pathological conditions. For example, systemic hypertension is associated with increased vascular stiffness, involving both the central (e.g., aorta, carotid) and peripheral (e.g., brachial, radial) vasculature [8-11,73]. Both increased distending pressure (passive effects) and structural alterations of the vessel wall (e.g., medial–intimal hypertrophy and hyperplasia, accumulation of collagen, elastin and mucopolysaccharides) are responsible for the increased stiffness. However, the relative contributions of the two factors may vary depending upon specific circumstances (e.g., age group, duration of hypertension, central vs. peripheral vasculature). In addition, structural bases for increased aortic wall stiffness in normal aging [7], atherosclerosis [14,15], and heritable disorders such as the Marfan Syndrome [74] are also well–defined. However, two important questions need to be addressed to evaluate the physiological relevance of quantifying aortic elastic properties: (1) How does increased aortic stiffness, independent of other cardiovascular factors, affect cardiovascular function? and (2) Is altered stiffness involved in the genesis and/or development/maintenance of the disease process or is it simply an obligatory consequence?

The first question may be addressed by considering three aspects of cardiovascular function: mechanical, energetic, and cardiovascular structural alterations. From the mechanical viewpoint, increased aortic stiffness (e.g., E_{inc}) results in increased aortic characteristic impedance (Z_c) and pulse wave velocity (*PWV*); although geometric changes (e.g., dilatation) can have offsetting effects [75]. Since Z_c is more sensitive to geometric changes [75], it is not uncommon to observe increased E_{inc} and *PWV* with unchanged Z_c when significant aortic dilatation is present. Finally, indices of wave reflections (e.g., magnitude of global reflection coefficient, Γ_G) would be either unchanged or increased depending upon the concomitant changes in systemic vascular resistance (*SVR*). Our recent experimental data [76], obtained in normal rabbit hearts, indicate that increased Z_c, *PWV*, and Γ_G all augment aortic pressure (P_{ao}) and flow (Q_{ao}) pulsatility (i.e., increased pulse pressure, narrow and tall flow pulse). However, *isolated* increments in Z_c, *PWV*, or Γ_G have only modest effects on systolic pressure (P_s) and stroke volume (*SV*) (< 6% increase in P_s and < 11% decrease in *SV* over a wide range of Z_c, *PWV*, and Γ_G). In contrast, diastolic pressure (P_d) is affected the most (up to 30% reduction over the same range). Thus, increased E_{inc} alone cannot result in selective and significant increase in P_s, such as that occurring in systolic hypertension. Consequently, other cardiovascular factors (e.g., increased *SVR*, LV end–diastolic volume and/or contractility) must coexist for systolic hypertension to develop. In summary, except for increased P_{ao} and Q_{ao} pulsatility and reduced P_d, the mechanical effects of increased E_{inc} in isolation are quite modest in the normal heart. Future studies are needed to examine if these observations hold true for a heart remodeled by long–term pressure and/or volume overload.

Changes in pulsatile arterial load, including aortic elastic properties, may also play a role in determining LV myocardial oxygen supply and demand (MVO_2). As discussed above, increments in large vessel stiffness cause diastolic pressures to fall and systolic pressures to rise, albeit by a small amount. A significant reduction in aortic diastolic pressure, a major determinant of coronary blood flow, may negatively impact on myocardial perfusion. This hemodynamic milieu would result in a decrease in oxygen supply at a time when MVO_2 may rise (secondary to the increase in systolic pressures). Kelly *et al.* [77] have shown that ejection into a stiff vascular system (i.e., increased aortic E_{inc}) does not change the intrinsic chemo–mechanical efficiency of normal hearts (i.e., MVO_2–PV area relationship). However, the $M\dot{V}O_2$ required to deliver a given cardiac output significantly increased (15%–41% increase). Since coronary flow reserve is often impaired in conditions with increased E_{inc} (e.g., systemic hypertension, atherosclerosis), it is likely that this increased MVO_2 may lead to supply–demand imbalance and myocardial ischemia.

Several pieces of relevant data can be cited indicating that pulsatile arterial load, including aortic elastic properties, is an independent determinant of left ventricular (LV) remodeling process. First, it has been shown that the application of static stress (strain) significantly increases protein synthesis in cell culture [78-81]. In addition, protein synthesis is further enhanced if the stress (strain) is applied in a pulsatile fashion [80]. Second, aortic pressure wave morphology appears to be related independently to LV mass. For example, even in the normotensive, normal population, late systolic rise in pressure (a characteristic of arterial stiffening) was associated with higher LV mass index [82]. Similarly, in a large population of non–hypertensive subjects, Darne *et al.* [83] have reported significant correlations between LV hypertrophy and both steady and pulsatile component indices of blood pressure. Safar and colleagues [84,85] found that for a given mean arterial pressure, cardiac mass was positively correlated with pulse pressure in middle–aged patients with systolic–diastolic hypertension. Fourth, different antihypertensive drugs that reduce mean blood pressure to the same extent do not regress LV hypertrophy by equivalent amounts [86]. It is possible that the differential responses of non–mechanical factors (i.e., neuro–humoral trophic stimuli) may be partially responsible for this observation. Thus, although the steady component of arterial load is the major mechanical determinant of LV remodeling, the role of pulsatile arterial load in this remodeling process may be more important than previously recognized. Finally, increased pulse pressure or cyclic stress has been postulated to accelerate the normal age–related remodeling of arterial wall (vessel dilatation and stiffening of the wall) [7,87] and to increase the susceptibility of vessel intima to atherosclerosis [88,89].

Since human data regarding aortic elastic properties are mostly derived from cross–sectional studies, limited information is available to address the second question posed above: Is altered arterial stiffness involved in the genesis and/or development/maintenance of the disease process or is it simply an obligatory consequence? Longitudinal data examining whether changes in aortic and large artery stiffness precede or follow the development of the disease process (e.g., systolic hypertension; the Marfan syndrome) are necessary to address this question. Clearly, only noninvasive techniques are suitable for this purpose.

Summary

Instantaneous aortic area measurements are greatly facilitated by the use of transesophageal echocardiography with automated border detection. The relative noninvasive nature of this technique is a clear advantage over other alternative invasive methods such as sonomicrometry, electrical calipers, and impedance catheter. In addition, measurements of aortic wall thickness can be readily obtained. When combined with noninvasive estimates of instantaneous aortic pressure, this technique allows serial assessment of aortic elastic properties. Such data may provide further insights into the pathophysiology of aging or disease states such as atherosclerosis, systemic hypertension and the Marfan syndrome. In addition, the long–term effects of antihypertensive agents on vascular elastic properties can be studied using these noninvasive techniques. This knowledge may help optimize the therapeutic strategy in individual patients.

Acknowledgments

We wish to acknowledge the valuable contributions of our colleagues Bernard P. Cholley, Claudia Korcarz, and David S. Berger.

References

1. Hallock P. Arterial elasticity in man in relation to age as evaluated by the pulse wave velocity method. *Arch Int Med* 1934;54:770-798.
2. Learoyd BM, Taylor MG. Alterations with age in the viscoelastic properties of human arterial walls. *Circ Res* 1966;18:278-292.
3. Gozna ER, Marbel AE, Shaw A, Holland JG. Age-related changes in the mechanics of the aorta and pulmonary artery of man. *J Appl Physiol* 1974;36:407-411.
4. Avolio AP, Deng FD, Li W, Lou Y, Huang Z, Zing L, O'Rourke MF. Effects of aging on arterial distensibility in populations with high and low prevalence of hypertension: comparison between urban and rural communities in China. *Circulation* 1984;71:202-210.
5. Kawasaki T, Sasayama S, Yagi SI, Asakama T, Hirai T. Noninvasive assessment of the age related changes in stiffness of major branches of the human arteries. *Cardiovasc Res* 1987;21:678-687.
6. Carroll JD, Shroff SG, Wirth P, Halsted M, Rajfer SI. Arterial mechanical properties in dilated cardiomyopathy: aging and the response to nitroprusside. *J Clin Invest* 1991;87:1002-1009.
7. O'Rourke MF. Effects of aging on aortic distensibility and aortic function in man. In: Boudoulas H, Toutouzas PK, Wooley CF, eds. *Functional Abnormalities of the Aorta*. Armonk, NY: Futura Publishing Company; 1996:279-293.
8. Safar ME, Toto-Moukouo JJ, Bouthier JA, Asmar RE, Levenson JA, Simon AC, London GM. Arterial dynamics, cardiac hypertrophy, and antihypertensive treatment. *Circulation* 1987;75 (Suppl I):I-156-I-161.
9. Laurent S, Lacolley P, London G, Safar M. Hemodynamics of the carotid artery after vasodilation in essential hypertension. *Hypertension* 1988;11:134-140.
10. O'Rourke MF. Arterial stiffness, systolic blood pressure, and logical treatment of arterial hypertension. *Hypertension* 1990;15:339-347.
11. Roman MJ, Pini R, Pickering TG, Devereux RB. Non-invasive measurements of arterial compliance in hypertensive compared with normotensive adults. *J Hypertens* 1992;10:S115-S118.
12. Yin FCP, Brin KP, Ting CT, Pyeritz RE. Arterial Hemodynamic Indexes in Marfan's Syndrome. *Circulation* 1989;79:854-862.
13. Hirata K, Triposkiadis F, Sparks E, Bowen J, Wooley C, Boudoulas H. The Marfan Syndrome: abnormal Aortic Elastic Properties. *J Am Coll Cardiol* 1991;18:57-63.
14. Farrar DJ, Green HD, Bond MG, Wagner WD, Gobbee RA. Aortic pulse wave velocity, elasticity, and composition in a nonhuman primate model of atherosclerosis. *Circ Res* 1978;43:52-62.
15. Farrar DJ, Bond MG, Riley WA, Sawyer JK. Anatomic correlates of aortic pulse wave velocity and carotid artery elasticity during atherosclerosis progression and regression in monkeys. *Circulation* 1991;83:1754-1763.
16. Atira T, Sasayama S, Kawasaki T, Tagi SI. Stiffness of systemic arteries in patients with myocardial infarction. *Circulation* 1989;80:78-86.

17. Stefanadis C, Wooley CF, Bush CA, Kolibash AJ, Boudoulas H. Aortic distensibility abnormalities in coronary artery disease. *Am J Cardiol* 1987;59:1300-1304.

18. Dart AM, Lacombe F, Yeoh JK, Cameron JD, Jennings JL, Laufer E, Esmore DS. Aortic distensibility in patients with isolated hypercholesterolemia, coronary artery disease, or cardiac transplant. *Lancet* 1991;338:270-273.

19. Arnett DK, Evans GW, Riley WA. Arterial stiffness: a new cardiovascular risk factor? *Am J Epidemiol* 1994;140:669-682.

20. O'Rourke MF, Taylor MG. Input impedance of the systemic circulation. *Circ Res* 1967;20:365-380.

21. McDonald DA: *Blood Flow in Arteries*. London, UK: Edward Arnold; 1974:351-388.

22. Milnor WR. Arterial impedance as ventricular afterload. *Circ Res* 1975;36:565-570.

23. Nichols WW, Pepine CJ, Geiser EA, Conti CR. Vascular load defined by the aortic input impedance spectrum. *Federation Proc* 1980;39:196-201.

24. O'Rourke MF. Vascular impedance in studies of arterial and cardiac function. *Physiol Rev* 1982;62:570-623.

25. Westerhof N, Elzinga G, Sipkema P. An artificial arterial system for pumping hearts. *J Appl Physiol* 1971;31:776-781.

26. Bourgeois MJ, Gilbert BK, Donald DE, Wood EH. Characteristics of aortic diastolic pressure decay with application to the continuous monitoring of changes in peripheral vascular resistance. *Circ Res* 1974;35:56-66.

27. Liu Z, Brin KP, Yin FCP. Estimation of total arterial compliance: an improved method and evaluation of current methods. *Am J Physiol* 1986;251:H588-H600.

28. Toorop GP, Westerhof N, Elzinga G. Beat-to-beat estimation of peripheral resistance and arterial compliance during pressure transients. *Am J Physiol* 1987;252:H1275-H1283.

29. Westerhof N, Sipkema P, Van den Bos GC, Elzinga G. Forward and backward waves in the arterial system. *Cardiovasc Res* 1972;6:648-656.

30. Lang RM, Cholley BP, Korcarz C, Marcus RH, Shroff SG. Measurements of regional elastic properties of the human aorta: a new application of transesophageal echocardiography with automated border detection and calibrated subclavian pulse tracings. *Circulation* 1994;90:1875-1882.

31. Patel DJ, De Freitas FM, Greenfield JC, Fry DL. Relationship of radius to pressure along the aorta in living dogs. *J Appl Physiol* 1963;18:1111-1117.

32. Gow BS, Taylor MG. Measurements of viscoelastic properties of arteries in the living dog. *Circ Res* 1968;23:111-122.

33. Pagani M, Schwartz PJ, Bishop VS, Malliani A. Reflex sympathetic changes in aortic diastolic pressure-diameter relationship. *Am J Physiol* 1975;229:286-290.

34. Pagani M, Mirksy I, Baig H, Thomas MW, Kerkhof P, Vatner SF. Effects of age on aortic pressure-diameter and elastic stiffness-stress relationships in unanesthetized sheep. *Circ Res* 1979;44:420-429.

35. Watkins RW, Sybertz EJ, Pula K, Antonellis A. Comparative effects of verapamil, diltiazem and nifedipine on aortic compliance in anesthetized dogs. *Arch Int Pharmacodyn* 1988;293:134-142.

36. Yano M, Kumada T, Matsuzaki M, Kohno M, Hiro T, Kohtoku S, Miura T, Katayama K, Ozaki M, Kusukawa R. Effect of diltiazem on aortic pressure-diameter relationship in dogs. *Am J Physiol* 1989;256:H1580-H1587.

37. Armentano RL, Levenson J, Barra JG, Fischer SIC, Breitbart GJ, Pichel RH, Simon A. Assessment of elastin and collagen contribution to aortic elasticity in conscious dogs. *Am J Physiol* 1991;260:H1870-H1877.

38. Barra JG, Armentano RL, Levenson J, Fischer EIC, Pichel RH, Simon A. Assessment of smooth muscle contribution to descending thoracic aortic elastic mechanics in conscious dogs. *Circ Res* 1993;73:1040-1050.

39. Wolinsky H, Glagov S. Structural basis for the static mechanical properties of the aortic media. *Circ Res* 1964;14:400-413.

40. Gozna ER, Marble AE, Shaw AJ, Winter DA. Mechanical properties of the ascending thoracic aorta of man. *Cardiovasc Res* 1973;7:261-265.

41. Stefanadis C, Stratos C, Boudoulas H, Kourouklis C, Toutouzas P. Distensibility of ascending aorta: comparison of invasive and non-invasive techniques in healthy men and in men with coronary artery disease. *Eur Heart J* 1990;11:990-996.

42. Ferguson JJ, Miller MJ, Sahagian P, Aroesty JM, McKay RG. Assessment of aortic pressure-volume relationships with an impedance catheter. *Cath Cardiovasc Diagn* 1988;15:27-36.

43. Stefanadis C, Boudoulas H, Toutouzas P. The aortic diameter-aortic pressure relationship in the clinical practice. In: Boudoulas H, Toutouzas PK, Wooley CF, eds. *Functional Abnormalities of the Aorta*. Armonk, NY: Futura Publishing Company; 1996:121-131.

44. Kohno M, Kumada T, Ozaki M, Matsuzaki M, Katayama K, Fujii T, Miura T, Kohtoki S, Yatabe S, Yano M, Hiro T, Kusukawa R. Evaluation of aortic wall distensibility by aortic pressure-dimension relation: effects of nifedipine on aortic wall. *Cardiovasc Res* 1987;21:305-312.

45. Steele JM. Interpretation of arterial elasticity from measurements of pulse wave velocity. *Am Heart J* 1937;12:452-464.

46. Latham RD, Westerhof N, Sipkema P, Rubal BJ, Reuderink BS, Murgo JP. Regional wave travel and reflections along the human aorta: a study with six simultaneous micromanometric pressures. *Circulation* 1985;72:1257-1269.

47. Safar ME, Perronneau PA, Levenson JA, Toto-Moukouo JA, Simon AC. Pulsed Doppler, diameter, blood flow velocity and volemic flow of the brachial artery in sustained essential hypertension. *Circulation* 1981;63:393-400.

48. Imura T, Yamamoto K, Kanamori K, Mikami T, Yasuda H. Noninvasive ultrasonic measurement of the elastic properties of the human abdominal aorta. *Cardiovasc Res* 1986;20:208-214.

49. Isnard RN, Pannier BM, Laurent S, London GM, Diebold B, Safar ME. Pulsatile diameter and elastic modulus of the aortic arch in essential hypertension: a noninvasive study. *J Am Coll Cardiol* 1989;13:399-405.

50. Mugge A, Daniel WG, Niedermeyer J, Hausman D, Nikutta P, Lichtlen PR. Usefulness of a new automatic boundary detection system for assesing stiffness of the descending thoracic aorta by transesophageal echocardiography. *Am J Cardiol* 1992;70:1629-1631.

51. Pasierski TJ, Binkley PF, Pearson AC. Evaluation of aortic distensibility with transesophageal echocardiography. *Am Heart J* 1992;123:1288-1292.

52. Perez JE, Waggoner AD, Barzilai B, Melton HE, Miller JG, Sobel BE. On-line assessment of ventricular function by automatic boundary detection and ultrasonic backscatter imaging. *J Am Coll Cardiol* 1992;19:313-320.

53. Perez JE, Klein SC, Prater DM, Fraser CE, Cardona H, Waggoner AD, Holland MR, Miller JG, Sobel BE. Automated on-line quantification of left ventricular dimensions and function by echocardiography with backscatter imaging and lateral gain compension. *Am J Cardiol* 1992;70:1200-1205.

54. Cholley BP, Shroff SG, Korcarz C, Lang RM. Aortic elastic properties with transesophageal echocardiography with automated border detection: validation according to regional differences between proximal and distal descending thoracic aorta. *J Am Soc Echocardiogr* 1996;9:539-548.

55. Bednarz JE, Marcus RH, Lang RM. Technical guidelines for performing automated border detection studies. *J Am Soc Echocardiogr* 1995;8:293-305.

56. Milnor WR. *Hemodynamics*. Baltimore, MD: Williams & Wilkins; 1989:58-101.

57. Slama MA, Fornes P, Heudes D, Diebold B, Fagon J, Safar ME. Measurement of aortic wall thickness by transesophageal echocardiography: an in-vitro validation. *J Am Coll Cardiol* 1994;23:145A (Abstract).

58. Marcus RH, Lang RM, Korcarz C, McCray G, Neuman A, Murphy M, Borow K, M., Weinert L, Bednarz J, Gretler DD, Sareli P. Noninvasive method for determination of arterial compliance using Doppler echocardiography and subclavian pulse tracings: validation and clinical application of a physiological model of the circulation. *Circulation* 1994;89:2688-2699.

59. Drzewiecki GM, Melbin J, Noordergraaf A. Arterial tonometry: review and analysis. *J Biomech* 1983;16:141-153.

60. Kelly R, Hayward C, Ganis J, Daley J, Avolio A, O'Rourke M. Noninvasive registration of the arterial pressure pulse waveform using high-fidelity applanation tonometry. *J Vasc Med Biol* 1989;1:142-149.

61. Kelly R, Karamanoglu M, Gibbs H, Avolio A, O'Rourke M. Non-invasive carotid pressure wave registration as an indicator of ascending aortic pressure. *J Vasc Med Biol* 1989;1:241-247.

62. Kelly R, Fitchett D. Noninvasive determination of aortic input impedance and external left ventricular power output: a validation and repeatability study of a new technique. *J Am Coll Cardiol* 1992;20:952-963.

63. Nichols WW, O'Rourke MF. *McDonald's Blood Flow in Arteries*. London, UK: Edward Arnold; 1990:216-250.

64. Shroff SG, Berger DS, Korcarz C, Lang RM, Marcus RH, Miller DE. Physiological relevance of T-tube model parameters with emphasis on arterial compliances. *Am J Physiol* 1995;269:H365-H374.

65. Horeman HW, Noordergraaf A. Numerical evaluation of volume pulsations in man: I. The basic formula. *Phys Med Biol* 1958;3:51-58.
66. Bergel DH. The static elastic properties of the arterial wall. *J Physiol* 1961;156:445-457.
67. Peterson L, Jensen RE, Parnel MS. Mechanical properties of arteries in vivo. *Circ Res* 1960;8:622-639.
68. Hayashi K, Handa H, Nagasawa S, Okumura A, Moritaki K. Stiffness and elastic behavior of human intracranial and extracranial arteries. *J Biomech* 1980;13:175-184.
69. Hirai T, Sasayama S, Kawasaki T, Yagi S. Stiffness of systemic arteries in patients with myocardial infarction: a new method to predict severity of coronary atherosclerosis. *Circulation* 1989;80:78-86.
70. Luchsinger PC, Sachs M, Patel DJ. Pressure-radius relationship in large blood vessels of man. *Circ Res* 1962;11:885-888.
71. Pieper HP, Paul LT. Responses of aortic smooth muscle studied in intact dogs. *Am J Physiol* 1969;217:154-160.
72. Patel DJ, Janicki JS, Carew TE. Static anisotropic elastic properties of the aorta in living dogs. *Circ Res* 1969;25:765-779.
73. Smulyan H, Vardan S, Griffiths A, Gribbin B. Forearm arterial distensibility in systolic hypertension. *J Am Coll Cardiol* 1984;3:387-393.
74. Perejda AJ, Abraham PA, Carnes WH, Coulson WF, Uitto J. Marfan syndrome: structural, biochemical, and mechanical studies of the aortic media. *J Lab Clin Med* 1985;106:376-383.
75. Noordergraaf A. *Circulatory System Dynamics*. New York, NY: Academic Press; 1978:105-156.
76. Berger DS, Robinson KA, Shroff SG. Wave propagation in the coupled left ventricle-arterial system: implications for aortic pressure. *Hypertension* 1996;27:1079-1089.
77. Kelly RP, Tunin R, Kass DA. Effect of reduced aortic compliance on cardiac efficiency and contractile function of in- situ canine left ventricle. *Circ Res* 1992;71:490-502.
78. Mann DL, Kent RL, Cooper G. Load regulation of the properties of adult feline cardiocytes: growth Induction by cellular deformation. *Circ Res* 1989;64:1079-1090.
79. Komuro I, Katoh Y, Kaida T, Shibazaki Y, Kurabayashi M, Hoh E, Takaku F, Yazaki Y. Mechanical loading stimulates cell hypertrophy and specific gene expression in cultured rat cardiac myocytes. *J Biol Chem* 1991;266:1265-1268.
80. McDonough PM, Glembotski CC. Induction of atrial natriuretic factor and myosin light chain-2 gene expression in cultured ventricular myocytes by electrical stimulation of contraction. *J Biol Chem* 1992;267:11665-11668.
81. Sadoshima J, Jahn L, Takahashi T, Kulik TJ, Izumo S. Molecular charactrization of the stretch-induced adaptation of cultured cardiac cells. *J Biol Chem* 1992;267:10551-10560.

82. Saba PS, Roman MJ, Pini R, Spitzer M, Ganau A, Devereux RB. Relation of arterial pressure waveform to left ventricular and carotid anatomy in normotensive subjects. *J Am Coll Cardiol* 1993;22:1873-1880.

83. Darne B, Girerd X, Safar M, Cambien F, Guize L. Pulsatile versus steady component of blood pressure: a cross-sectional analysis and a prospective analysis on cardiovascular mortality. *Hypertension* 1989;13:392-400.

84. Safar ME, Laurent S, Safavian AL, Pannier BM, London GM. Pulse pressure in sustained essential hypertension: a hemodynamic study. *J Hypertens* 1987;5:213-218.

85. Safar ME. Pulse pressure in essential hypertension: clinical and therapeutical implications. *J Hypertens* 1989;7:769-776.

86. Dahlof B, Pennert K, Hansson L. Reversal of left ventricular hypertrophy in hypertensive patients. *Am J Hypertens* 1992;5:95-110.

87. O'Rourke MF. Basic concepts for the understanding of large arteries in hypertension. *J Cardiovasc Pharmacol* 1985;7:S-14-S-21.

88. Johnson WTM, Salanga G, Lee GA, Himelstein AL, Wall SJ, Horwitz O. Arterial intimal embrittlement. A possible factor in atherogesis. *Arteriosclerosis* 1986;59:161-171.

89. Glagov S, Grande JP, Xu C-P, Giddens DP, Zarins CK. Limited effects of hyperlipidemia on the arterial smooth muscle response to mechanical stress. *J Cardiovasc Pharmacol* 1989;14:S-90-S-97.

7 Left Atrial Function: Indirect Hemodynamic Assessment Using Acoustic Quantification

Alan D. Waggoner and Julio E. Pérez

The importance of left atrial (LA) size and function has been recognized in variety of clinical conditions including embolic stroke, atrial fibrillation, hypertension, acute myocardial infarction and mitral regurgitation. Indirect atrial assessment of LA function during cardiac catheterization includes measurements of pulmonary capillary wedge pressure or left ventricular (LV) end diastolic pressure (LVEDP) but rarely involves direct measurement of LA pressure or performance of LA angiography. Noninvasively, LA size and function can be assessed by M-Mode or two dimensional (2D) echo-cardiography and, indirectly, via pulsed Doppler echocardiographic measurements of mitral inflow and pulmonary venous flow velocities. Limitations of these methods include their indirect nature and that only a few cardiac cycles are usually analyzed. Real time, on-line boundary detection with 2D echocardiography, commercialized as Acoustic Quantification (AQ), has been shown to provide quantitative analysis of LA size and function. This chapter focuses on invasive and noninvasive measurements of LA function and applications of AQ for the assessment of LA performance and the future potential of AQ in clinical situations.

The Concept of LA Function

LA function has been traditionally defined as comprising two components, filling and emptying. During ventricular systole, the left atrium functions as a reservoir via pulmonary venous inflow, or through the mitral valve when mitral regurgitation is present. Despite clinical situations where enlargement of the LA occurs, systolic pulmonary venous flow continues uninterrupted unless there is severe mitral regurgitation [1], markedly elevated LA pressure or atrial fibrillation. After mitral valve opening, at the onset of diastole, LA emptying begins as a conduit for pulmonary venous flow to augment early LV filling. In late diastole, active atrial contraction occurs in sinus rhythm (often considered the booster pump function) completing the ventricular filling. Grant *et al.* [2] established the importance of the "reservoir" function of the LA in 23 patients using simultaneous invasive measurements of LA pressure and angiography to construct pressure-volume loops. This initial report concluded that systolic filling of the LA was of greater importance in LV filling than atrial contraction, except in patients with left ventricular hypertrophy.

Hemodynamic variables influence LA emptying, particularly LVEDP. Wallace and co-workers reported that increasing heart rate alone led to increased LA pressure without changes in LVEDP [3]. Although one may speculate that a close relationship would exist between mean LA volume and mean pressure, Sauter and co-workers [4] found no direct relationship between LA volume and pressure in patients with mitral stenosis or regurgitation. There was a reasonable linear correlation (r=0.86) in patients with dilated cardiomyopathy or aortic stenosis. Stott *et al.* [5] established the importance of active LA contraction in patients with aortic stenosis, compared to those with mitral stenosis. This was evident despite higher mean LA pressures in mitral valve disease but higher LVEDP in patients with aortic stenosis. The LV shape, wall thickness and size, representing components of LV compliance during late diastole, also had an influential role in LA mechanics. This is particularly evident in the hypertrophied LV where in early diastole the LA-LV pressure difference is minimal, while in late diastole the LV pressure-volume relationship is steeper. In this setting a forceful atrial contraction is necessary to augment LV volume unless there is elevated mean LA pressure due to heart failure. Rahimtoola and co-workers [6] extended these observations and reported the importance of active LA contraction in patients with previous myocardial infarction and its effect on LVEDP and volume. The contribution of LA contraction to LVEDP and LV volume was greater in patients post MI relative to normal controls. The LA contribution was less in patients with enlarged LV volumes than in those with normal LV end-diastolic volumes. However, in the setting of a low cardiac output state, the contribution of LA contraction was most pronounced. Hitch and Noonan [7] studied components of LA reservoir, conduit and pump function and concluded that heart rate, end-diastolic length of ventricular fibers and the relationship of atrial systole and ventricular systole all have an influence on LA function. The LA reservoir function was present to a minor extent even during early diastole, while LA booster pump function varied directly with reservoir function. As the reservoir or the booster pump function of the LA increases the conduit function decreases.

Alteration in hemodynamics due to increased catecholamines, autonomic stimulation (or depression) or volume loading influence LA function similarly to the effects on LV function. Payne and colleagues [8] demonstrated in an animal model (using sonomicrometer crystals implanted in the LA wall) that the LA diameter increased with volume loading as did atrial contraction while the LA pressure remained normal. However, with further increases in LA size there was loss of atrial contractility and LA pressure continued to increase while the conduit function of the LA was actually enhanced. Williams *et al.* [9] evaluated atrial force in experimental animals using length-tension curves during a variety of interventions. Atrial function was enhanced by stimulation of the right vagus nerve or by changes induced by positive inotropic agents (isoproterenol, calcium, or acetyl-strophanthidin) but depressed when the left vagus nerve was stimulated or aortic pressures were increased. Thus, the Frank-Starling mechanism operates in atrial myocardium similar to the case of ventricular myocardium. There is relatively equal force generated by each chamber when differences in mass are taken into consideration. As LA dilatation occurs the active LA contractile function becomes depressed.

Hemodynamic Studies Related to LA Function

Recently, there has been a renewed interest in LA function derived from studies that have employed hemodynamic data obtained in the cardiac catheterization laboratory. These studies have further increased our understanding of LA-LV interaction. Matsuzaki *et al.* [10] evaluated LA pump function in controls, in patients with remote myocardial infarction and in patients with arterial hypertension using simultaneous LA pressure (by catheter tip manometer) and M-Mode recordings of the LA and posterior aortic wall motion to derive pressure-dimension loops. The peak tension (product of LA pressure and LA dimension during active contraction) was higher in the patients, as was LA diameter, compared to controls. The LA work was increased with augmented preload in patients with remote infarction or due to an enhanced inotropic state in those with arterial hypertension. These authors reported in another study [11] that although LA contractility, derived from LA angiographic volume studies with simultaneously measured pressure, was similar in patients with coronary artery disease and controls, patients with coronary artery disease exhibited increased LA work. There was also an inverse relationship between LV ejection fraction and LA work.

Sanada and co-workers [12] studied patients with either hypertension or hypertrophic cardiomyopathy and determined that LA afterload mismatch was apparent, with higher LA stroke work in patients with hypertension but there was impaired LA active contraction in patients with hypertrophic cardiomyopathy. There was a inverse relationship between LA stroke index and the LV chamber stiffness constant. Sigwart *et al.* [13] studied patients undergoing percutaneous transluminal angioplasty and reported increases in LA maximal and stroke volumes during atrial contraction despite marked increases in LA mean pressure. This was observed in all 10 patients but without accompanying changes in heart rate. In contrast to the work of Sauter *et al.*, Sigwart and co-workers noted changes in LA pressure during myocardial ischemia directly correlated with changes in LA volume. Most of the patients had normal LA volumes prior to angioplasty, however no mention was made as to if mitral regurgitation was present.

Sasayama *et al.*, in an experimental study [14], created mitral regurgitation of varying severity in dogs while measuring changes in LA diameters (measured with ultrasonic crystals) and LA pressure. With induction of moderate MR, the LA pressure and diameter increased as did LA active shortening. With severe MR, the LA diameter increased further while LA active shortening diminished significantly. Afterload reduction, in the setting of severe MR however, decreased LA size and improved LA shortening by 50%. The decrease in LA contractile function in acute, severe MR may have been related to overstretching of atrial myocardium in the descending limb of the Frank-Starling curve and the increased afterload from elevated LA and LV end diastolic pressures. The LA compliance (reservoir function) was impaired in these studies due to increasing severity of MR that was accompanied by marked elevations in LA pressure but without significant changes in LA diameters.

These investigators also performed a follow-up study using a chronic MR experimental animal model [15]. The LA stroke work index increased as did LA size but without loss of LA shortening such as was observed in the acute model. Interestingly, the LA compliance was actually enhanced in chronic MR and reservoir function was maintained. This was observed however without increases in LA pressure in the early to late follow-up period. The LA wall thickness measured at necropsy was found to be slightly increased.

Noninvasive Assessment of LA Function

Initial studies of LA function were carried out with M-Mode and two dimensional (2D) echocardiographic assessment of LA size or volumes. Loperfido *et al.* [16] found an excellent correlation (r=0.90) between 2D measured LA volume (area-length method) and LA angiography. Schabelmann *et al.* [17] compared both M-Mode and 2D estimations of volume to LA volume derived angiographically (during levophase portion of pulmonary artery contrast injections) and found that combining 2D apical-4 and 2-chamber views with the method of discs provided the best correlation with invasively-derived volume. Later work, from the same institution, evaluated LA function in normal volunteers [18]. Their results disclosed the normal LA end systolic volume was 37±12 ml and decreased by 24±8 ml at end diastole with a calculated emptying fraction of 65±9%. Gehr *et al.* [19] noted similar values in 9 normal patients. The values of maximal LA volume by 2D echocardiography from both of these studies are however lower than previously reported [20] angiographic volumes in normals (63±16 ml) while the fractional emptying index is slightly higher with echocardiography (angiographic = 52±17%). Hofstetter *et al.* [21] evaluated healthy infants and children to derive 2D echocardiographic estimated LA volumes and fractional emptying index and found these parameters to be comparable to these of adults.

The role of the mitral annulus descent and LA function was evaluated by Jones *et al.* [22] using M-Mode recordings of standard parasternal LA size and measurements obtained from the base of the mitral valve to the posterior aspect of the LA in apical 4-chamber view. During ventricular systole the apical descent of the mitral annulus is accompanied by increases in LA size in the transverse plane thought to be responsible for facilitating pulmonary venous flow and atrial reservoir function. During early ventricular diastole, the motion of the mitral annulus back towards the LA presumably occurs due to elastic forces in the atrial wall using stored energy derived from ventricular myocardium. The motion of the mitral annulus during late diastole was observed also to play a role in atrial systolic function. This was the first study to show that LA-LV interaction can be evaluated with 2D echocardiographic imaging.

The relationship between LA size and function to LVEDP was evaluated by Appleton *et al.* [23]. Both maximal and minimal LA volumes were higher in patients with elevated pulmonary wedge (>12 mmHg) and elevated LV EDP compared to those with normal values. The LA emptying fraction was lower in patients with elevated, as compared to those with normal LVEDP (32±15% vs 55±10%). The LA emptying fraction was correlated with pulmonary wedge pressure (r=0.70) and with LVEDP (r=0.70). Patients with MR or mitral stenosis were excluded from this study and there were no differences in LV ejection fraction between patients with elevated and normal LVEDP. Therefore increased LA size and reduced active LA contractile function was associated with increased LVEDP due to LV diastolic dysfunction.

Measurements of LA volumes and emptying fraction by two dimensional echocardiography have also been reported in patients with mitral valve disease. Gehr *et al.* [19] performed frame by frame analysis of LA volumes employing the apical-4-chamber view and calculated fractional emptying indexes in normals and in patients with mitral valve disease. As expected LA volumes were increased in patients with severe MR, and in those with mitral stenosis whether the rhythm was sinus or atrial fibrillation. The LA emptying fraction (maximal-minimal/maximal volume) was reduced in most of the patients. Ren *et al.* [24] noted that a LA emptying volume >40 ml was always observed in patients with moderate or severe MR. Therefore, a larger LA volume would have been associated with a higher emptying volume but two dimensional echocardiographic evaluation does not account for the contribution of pulmonary venous inflow during the conduit phase of the LA emptying.

Indirect measurements of LA function employing pulsed Doppler of mitral inflow and pulmonary venous flow velocities complement imaging of the LA size and provide information regarding conduit function and active atrial contraction. Since LA dilatation due to volume (or pressure) overload ultimately leads to depression of atrial function, when LA pressure is elevated, it is expected to induce a reduction in A wave amplitude of mitral inflow velocities. Alternatively, enhanced atrial contraction in conditions of increased heart rate, myocardial ischemia or ventricular hypertrophy result in higher A wave velocities. Pulmonary venous flow patterns are also influenced by LA reservoir function. There is blunted systolic pulmonary venous flow in conditions of reduced LA function (*i.e.* atrial fibrillation) as well as augmented systolic flow when active LA contraction is enhanced. However Doppler parameters based on pulmonary venous flow and mitral inflow velocities are related to the instantaneous LA-LV pressure difference during diastole and provide little information regarding LA reservoir function.

On-Line Evaluation of LA Function Using Acoustic Quantification

On-line detection of LA size using Acoustic Quantification (AQ) and function has relied upon LA imaging from the apical 4-chamber view (Figure 7.1).

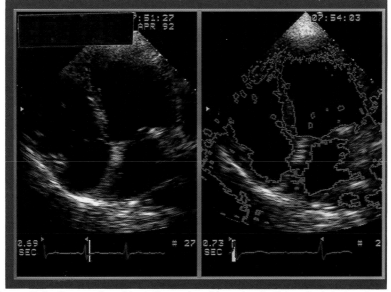

Figure 7.1. Conventional two dimensional imaging in the apical 4 chamber view in left panel and boundary detection image in the right panel.

Lateral gain controls are usually employed to improve detection of the atrial septum and lateral walls of the left atrium (Figure 7.2).

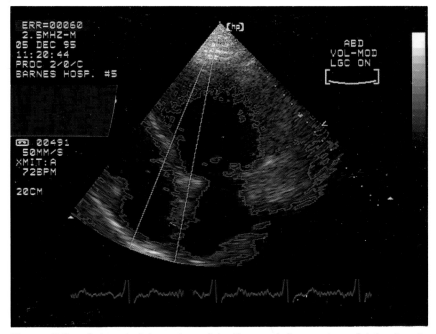

Figure 7.2. Automated boundary detection and the sector of lateral gain compensation to enhance borders of the atrial septum.

Time gain compensation must be also carefully adjusted to obtain images of the LA chamber without gain artifacts and to prevent overlap of signals from the LV. The ultrasound imaging system allow the operator to quickly switch back and forth from AQ to conventional imaging. This is necessary to verify that the on-line boundary detection algorithm is accurately tracking the LA borders.

Once accurate border detection is verified, the operator proceeds to place the region-of-interest (point-to-point tracing or circled-area methods) in real time around the LA blood pool (Figure 7.3). The region of interest is positioned across the mitral annulus at end-diastole to avoid including the LV blood pool area. Alternatively the operator can increase the time gain compensation setting at the level of the mitral annulus to create a boundary at that level. After positioning the region of interest, the operator selects the atrial area waveform software display which depicts the instantaneous changes in LA area simultaneously with the electrocardiogram and real time 2D imaging (Figure 7.3).

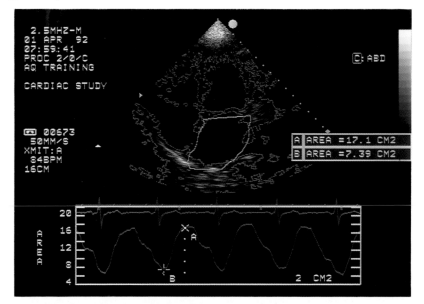

Figure 7.3. Quantification of left atrial area by automated boundary detection in the same patient as in Figure 7.1. The end systolic area (caliper A) was 17.1 cm² and end diastolic area (caliper B) was 7.4 cm² (fractional area change 57%).

By including the major or axis length of the LA one can obtain volumetric data displayed in real time by either area-length or method of disc approximation (Figure 7.4).

We and others have validated the accuracy of on-line AQ for assessment of LA area and function when compared to conventional 2D derived areas [25,26]. Our initial study included 55 patients, 35 of whom were in sinus rhythm, 10 in atrial fibrillation and 10 normal volunteers studied as controls. Moderate to severe MR was present in 16 of the patients. Both LA minimal (at end diastole) and maximal (at end systole, just before mitral valve opening) cavity areas by the on-line method demonstrated excellent correlation's with LA areas obtained by off-line measurement of conventional 2D imaging (r=0.91 and 0.93, respectively). In normal subjects the LA areas at end diastole were 7.8±2.4 cm² and 13.6 ± 2.7 cm² at end systole. The normal LA emptying index was 44±0.09% and was derived as end-systolic area minus end-diastolic area divided by end-systolic area. The normal LA expansion index was 81±32% and was calculated as end-systolic area minus end-diastolic area divided by end-diastolic area.

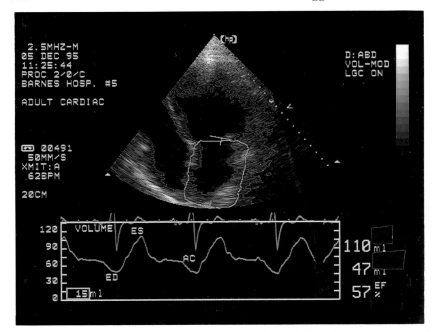

Figure 7.4. Automated boundary detection of the left atrial volume at end diastole (ED) of 47 ml and end systole (ES) of 110 ml by the area length method. The emptying fraction (EF) was 57%. Note the period of diastasis and decrease in volume with atrial contraction (AC).

Patients with MR had larger LA cavity areas and lower LA emptying index than those without MR. Most patients in our study however had reduced LA fractional emptying (even those without MR) and nearly all had LV dysfunction. Also the LA emptying index was significantly lower in patients with atrial fibrillation as compared to those in sinus rhythm (0.28 ± 0.12 vs 0.17 ± 0.05, $p<0.02$). Thus, LA function, as assessed by on-line AQ, is abnormal in patients with chronic MR and in those with atrial fibrillation. Coexistent LV systolic dysfunction may also be responsible for the lower values of LA emptying in these patients.

The initial studies with on-line derived LA area and function have been extended in additional studies [27]. This has included patients evaluated after the Maze surgical procedure to treat patients with chronic atrial fibrillation [28], patients evaluated after cardiac transplantation [29] and patients evaluated for LA appendage function in sinus rhythm or in atrial fibrillation [30]. All of these patient groups exhibit abnormalities in LA function which have been evaluated previously with pulsed Doppler echocardiography. The Maze procedure is a recently developed surgical technique to correct atrial fibrillation. On-line AQ of the left atrium was used to evaluate LA function in 25 patients an average of 6 ± 2 months after surgery and results were compared to age-matched normal controls [28]. All patients following the Maze procedure exhibited increased LA areas. There were 21 patients (84%) who exhibited restored, but depressed active (late-diastolic) atrial function as measured by percent atrial contribution as compared to controls ($10\pm6\%$ vs $24\pm16\%$; $p<0.001$). The LA conduit function (diastolic emptying prior to atrial contraction) was similar, however LA expansion was decreased in the patients relative to controls. Although LA function remains impaired in these patients at short term follow-up, none of the patients have experienced adverse clinical events. These findings are not unexpected since direct current cardioversion for atrial fibrillation is also associated with impaired atrial function, (as measured by Doppler echocardiography) in most patients following successful restoration of electrical atrial activity. The duration of atrial fibrillation and LA enlargement are probably key factors in the successful recovery of LA function in this instance.

Patients who underwent orthotopic cardiac transplantation may have altered atrial function as the donor and recipient atrial components exhibit dyssynchronous activation as detected by surface electrocardiography. We evaluated 20 clinically stable patients (without allograft rejection criteria) at 3.5 ± 0.3 (SE) years following transplantation with on-line AQ indices of LA function [29]. A unique aspect of the study was the ability to localize the region of interest to either the donor or recipient portions of the LA in addition to the entire LA from two-dimensional images (Figure 7.5).

Measurements were made of LA size and function with particular interest to the active contraction phase of each portion of the LA (donor, recipient, global). The apical 4-chamber view was obtained and the visualized suture line served as the demarcation between donor and recipient regions of the LA. All patients had normal global and segmental LV systolic performance. Global LA area, emptying fraction and percent area change due to atrial contraction was significantly lower in transplant patients as compared to measurements obtained from controls. When the individual components of the transplanted LA were analyzed, the donor portion accounted for most of active late-diastolic contraction while the recipient component exhibited virtually no active contraction. In some patients the recipient portion actually expanded during atrial systole. Pulsed Doppler recording of mitral inflow velocities (E early ventricular filling, A: atrial contraction; isovolumic relaxation and mitral deceleration times) were obtained in all patients. All patients had increased E/A ratios (mean 2.2), normal E velocity (mean: 76 cm/s) and borderline increased isovolumic relaxation times (mean: 88 ms) with borderline shortened deceleration times (mean 167 ms). We postulated that the observed increase in mitral valve E/A ratio by Doppler was primarily a result of left atrial dysfunction (blunting the A wave velocity) rather than due to restrictive ventricular physiology as the LVEDP was normal in all patients in whom it was measured in separate catheterization studies.

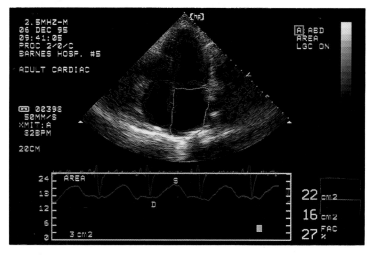

Figure 7.5(A). Apical four-chamber view using automated boundary detection and region of interest encompassing the entire left atrium in a patient following orthotopic heart transplantation. The maximal systolic (S) area is 22 cm² and the end diastolic (D) area is 16 cm². The fractional area change (FAC) from end-systole to end-diastole is 27%.

The application of on-line AQ to assess LA size and LA appendage function in patients with sinus rhythm or atrial fibrillation was recently reported by Rosen *et al.* [30]. The LA size and LA appendage was larger in those with atrial fibrillation. However, the fractional area change of the LA appendage was greater in patients with sinus rhythm. Maximal atrial contraction occurred after the P wave of the electrocardiogram corresponding to the timing of maximal atrial contraction of the LA chamber (the LA emptying fraction was not measured in this study).

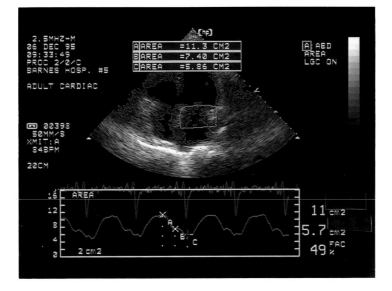

Figure 7.5(B). Apical four-chamber view using automated boundary detection and region of interest drawn around the donor portion of the left atrium in the same patient as Figure 5A. Caliper A is the end systolic area of 11 cm² , caliper B is the end diastolic area of 7.4 cm² and caliper C is the end diastolic area of 5.86 cm². The fractional area change (FAC) is 49%. Note the smaller area change of 1.5 cm² from mid diastole to end diastole.

The delineation of LA pressure-area loops with AQ was described by Keren *et al.* [31-33] in an experimental animal model. Simultaneous measurements of LA pressure and LA area by AQ exhibited an increase during systole and a decrease during passive LA emptying. Increased LA pressure resulted in impaired atrial contraction by on-line AQ recording of LA area from apical 4-chamber view, but not from a parasternal long axis views. Experimental induction of MR led to increases in LA pressure and LA area with enhanced rate of change of LA area (dA/dt) during LA filling and passive emptying, despite increases in the LA stiffness constant. The authors pointed out the feasibility of obtaining the LA pressure-volume loops. However, the method does have certain limitations [33]. Most notably this relates to the inherent delay in the AQ display of LA area relative to pressure change which ranged from 20-34 ms, limiting the true simultaneous recording of events. This delay was greater (35-57 ms) at lower frame rates (30 Hz vs 60 Hz). Further work will be necessary with correction for the time delays in the graphic recordings of AQ derived LA area relative to the instantaneous LA pressure.

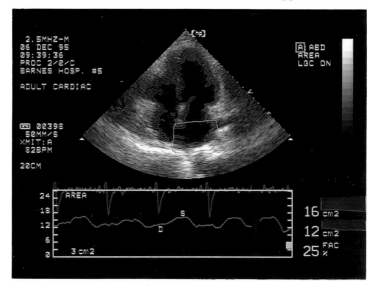

Figure 7.5(C). Apical four-chamber view with automated boundary detection and region of interest drawn around the recipient LA as in the previous figure. The maximal end systolic area (s) is 16 cm² and the end diastolic area (D) is 12 cm² with a fractional area change during diastole of 25%.

Limitations of On-Line AQ Measurements

Another obvious difficulty with on-line AQ measurements of LA size and functional characteristics relate to the limitations of conventional 2D image quality. For example the relative contribution of the atrial septum to LA function is likely negligible but detection of the atrial septum with automated boundary detection is often difficult, such as when it is displaced or oscillates during the cardiac cycle as seen in cases of atrial septal aneurysm. Measurements of LA area by on-line AQ correlate well with conventional echocardiographic and sonomicrometer crystals data but the accuracy of LA volume determination by on-line AQ will require further correlative studies. The use of other views such as parasternal long, or short axis view, or the apical two-chamber with respect to obtaining accurate functional parameters of LA area, volume and function are yet to be established.

Future Directions

The influence of inotropic stimulation (*i.e.* dobutamine) on LA function will be of interest to ascertain its effect on LA size, with respect to reservoir function or active atrial emptying. Abnormalities in atrial conduction such as first degree atrioventricular (AV) block or optimal programming of AV sequential pacemakers might be applicable to on-line AQ derived perimeters of LA function. Further work will be needed to assess changes in LA size and the effect on parameters of LA function (such as in the expansion index) absence of MR in patients with LV dysfunction. Comparison with Doppler parameters of maximal or mean atrial velocity, duration of flow velocity and pulmonary venous inflow characteristics will be also necessary. The relationship between LA function, pressure and mitral or pulmonary venous flow velocities or LV function are of continuing interest with regards to LA-LV coupling.

Conclusions

The LA size and function can be assessed accurately in most patients with on-line AQ derived area or volume, including the rates of area change per unit time. The unique contribution of AQ to study LA function in patients following surgical correction of atrial fibrillation and evaluation of regional function after cardiac transplantation have been highlighted. AQ provides direct and complementary information to the indirect Doppler assessment via recordings mitral inflow velocities to assess LA reservoir, conduit and active emptying functional parameters. Further work regarding its role the assessment of LA-LV coupling remains to be carried out and in a variety of clinical settings.

References

1. Braunwald E, Frahm CJ: Studies on Starling's law of the heart. IV. Observations on the hemodynamic function of the left atrium in man. *Circulation* 1961;24:633-642.
2. Grant C, Bunnell IL, Greene DG: The reservoir function of the left atrium during ventricular systole. An angiographic study of atrial stroke volume and work. *Am J Med* 1964;37:36-43.
3. Wallace AG, Mitchell JH, Skinner NS, Sarnoff SJ: Hemodynamic variables affecting the relation between mean left atrial and left ventricular end diastolic pressures. *Circ Res* 1963;13:261-270.
4. Sauter HJ, Dodge HT, Johnston RR, Graham TP: The relationship of left atrial pressure and volume in patients with heart disease. *Am Heart J* 1964;67:635-642.

5. Stott DK, Marpole DGF, Bristow JD, Kloster FE, Griswold HE: The role of left atrial transport in aortic and mitral stenosis. *Circulation* 1970;41:1031-1041.
6. Rahimtoola SH, Ehsani A, Sinno MZ, Loeb HS, Rosen KM, Gunnar RM: Left atrial transport function in myocardial function. Importance of its booster pump function. *Am J Med* 1975;59:686-693.
7. Hitch DC, Nolan SP: Descriptive analysis of instantaneous left atrial volume-with special reference to left atrial function. *J Surg Research* 1981;30:110-120.
8. Payne RM, Stone HL, Engelken EJ: Atrial function during volume loading. *J Applied Physiol* 1971;31:326-331.
9. Williams JF Jr., Sonnenblick EH, Braunwald E: Determinants of atrial contractile force in the intact heart. *Am J Physiol* 1965;209:1061-1068.
10. Matsuzaki M, Tamitani M, Toma Y, Ogawa H, Latayama K, Matsuda Y, Kusukawa R: Mechanism of augmented left atrial pump function in myocardial infarction and essential hypertension evaluated by left atrial pressure-dimension relation. *Am J Cardiol* 1991;67:1121-1126.
11. Matsuda Y, Toma Y, Ogawa H, Matsuzaki M, Katayama K, Fujii T, Yoshino F, Maritani K, Kumada T, Kusukawa R: Importance of left atrial function in patients with myocardial infarction. *Circulation* 1983;67:566-571.
12. Sanada H, Shimizu M, Shimizu K, Kita Y, Sugihara N, Takeda R: Left atrial afterload mismtach in hypertrophic cardiomyopathy. *Am J Cardiol* 1991;68:1049-1054.
13. Sigwart U, Grbic M, Goy JJ, Kappenberger L: Left atrial function in acute transient left ventricular ischemia produced during percutaneous transluminal coronary angioplasty of the left anterior descending coronary artery. *Am J Cardiol* 1990;65:282-286.
14. Sasayama S, Takahashi M, Osakada G, Hirose K, hamashima H, Nishimura E, Kawai C: Dynamic geometry of the left atrium and left ventricle in acute mitral regurgitation. *Circulation* 1979;60:177-186.
15. Kihara Y, Sasayama S, Miyazaki S, Onodera T, Susawa T, Nakamura Y, Fujiwara H, Kawai C: Role of the left atrium in adaptation of the heart to chronic mitral regurgitation in conscious dogs. *Circ Res* 1988;62:543-553.
16. Loperfido F, Pennestri F Digaetano A, Scablia E, Santarelli P, Mongiardo R, Schiavoni G, Cappola E, Manzoli U: Assessment of left atrial dimension by cross-sectional echocardiography in patients with mitral valve disease. *Br Heart J* 1983;50:570-577.
17. Schabelman S, Schiller NB, Silverman NH, Ports TA: Left atrial volume estimation by two dimensional echocardiography. *Cathet Cardiovasc Diagn* 1981;7:165-178.
18. Gutman J, Wang YS, Wahr D, Schiller NB: Normal left atrial function determined by two dimensional echocardiography. *Am J Cardiol* 1983;51:336-340.
19. Gehr LG, Mintz GS, Kotler MN, Segal BL: Left atrial volume overload in mitral regurgitation: A two dimensional echocardiographic study. *Am J Cardiol* 1982;49:33-38.
20. Murray JA, Kennedy JW, Figley MW: Quantitative angiocardiography. II. The normal left atrial volume in man. *Circulation* 1968;37:800-804.

21. Hofstette5r R, Bartz-Bazzanella P, Kentrup H, Von Bermuth G: Determination of left atrial area and volume by cross-sectional echocardiography in healthy infants and children. *Am J Cardiol* 1991;68:1073-1078.

22. Jones CJH, Song GJ, Gibson DG: An echocardiographic assessment of atrial mechanical behaviour. *Br Heart J* 1991;65:31-36.

23. Appleton CP, Galloway JM, Gonzalez MS, Gaballa M, Basnight MA: Estimation of left ventricular filling pressures using two dimensional and Doppler echocardiography in adult patients with cardiac disease. Additional value of analyzing left atrial size, left atrial ejection fraction and the difference in duration of pulmonary venous and mitral flow velocity at atrial contraction. *J Am Coll Cardiol* 1993;22:1972-1982.

24. Ren JF, Kotter MN, De Pace NL: Two dimensional echocardiographic determination of left atrial emptying volume: A non-invasive index in quantifying the degree of nonrheumatic mitral regurgitation. *J Am Coll Cardiol* 1983;2:729-736.

25. Waggoner AD, Barzilai B, Miller JG, Perez JE: On line assessment of left atrial area and function by echocardiographic automatic boundary detection. *Circulation* 1993;88:1142-1149.

26. Foster E, Barbant SD, Schiller NB: Automated border detection of left atrial size: On-line measurements of time-area relationships. *J Am Soc Echocardiogr* 1992;5:334 (Abstract).

27. Athanassopoulos G, Karatasakis G, Cokkinos DV: Relation between atrial function evaluated with two dimensional echocardiography with automatic border detection and relevant atrioventricular diastolic flow dynamics. *Eur Heart J* 1993;14:225 (Abstract).

28. Feinberg MS, Waggoner AD, Kater KM, Cox JL, Perez JE: Echocardiographic automatic boundary detection to measure left atrial function after the Maze procedure. *J Am Soc Echocardiogr* 1995;8:139-148.

29. Cresci S, Goldstein JM, Cardona H, Waggoner AD, Perez JE: Impaired left atrial function after heart transplantation: Disparate contribution of donor and recipient atrial components studied on-line with quantitative echocardiography. *J Heart Lung Transplant* 1995;14:647-653.

30. Rosen SE, Baruch L, Vorchheimer DA, Fisher EA, Budd J, David O, Rosenthal M, Goldman ME: Left atrial appendage function in atrial fibrillation: Assessment with transesophageal echocardiographic on-line automated border detection system. *J Am Coll Cardiol* 1994;282A (Abstract).

31. Keren A, DeAnda A, Komeda M, Tye T, Daughters GT, Ingels NB, Miller C, Popp RL, Nikolic SD: Left atrial pressure-area relationship obtained by automated border detection. *J Am Soc Echcoardiogr* 1994;7:S42 (Abstract).

32. Keren A, DeAnda A, Komeda M, Tye T, Daughters GT, Nikolic SD: Automated border detection in evaluaton of left atrial area and stiffness. *Circulation* 1994;90:I-598 (Abstract).

33. Keren A, DeAnda A, Komeda M, Tye T, Handen CE, Daughters GT, Ingels NB, Miller C, Popp RL: Pitfalls in creation of left atrial pressure-area relationships with automated border detection. *J Am Soc Echocardiogr* 1995;8:669-678.

8 On-line Quantification Of Cardiovascular Function In Children

Thomas R. Kimball

On-line quantification of ventricular performance using automated border detection is ideally suited for application in the pediatric population. Typically, the echocardiographic image quality in children is excellent enabling endocardial definition throughout the cardiac cycle. In addition this technique is readily applicable to pediatric cardiovascular issues that traditionally have been difficult to assess using current methodologies. For example, evaluation of ventricular function in chambers with unusual geometry (*i.e.* single ventricles) can now be assessed using this technique. It also provides a relatively easy, and perhaps more accurate, method of evaluating ventricular diastolic function. It may also allow noninvasive diagnosis of transplant rejection, a clinically vexing problem that has traditionally required endomyocardial biopsy. Most promising, pediatric cardiologists can now explore new issues such as developmental changes in arterial vasoreactivity and ventricular-arterial coupling with automated quantification methods employing noninvasive ultrasound.

Clinical Uses of Acoustic Quantification in Children

General Considerations

The technologic evolution of echocardiography has been rapid and dramatic. Initially, pediatric cardiologists relied solely on M-mode echocardiography.

The unidimensional, "ice-pick view" of the heart offered by M-mode echocardiography limited the ability to image cardiac anatomy. Recently, pediatric cardiologists have witnessed extraordinary advances as two-dimensional, Doppler, and color Doppler echocardiography have been developed. These modalities have resulted in the unprecedented ability to image cardiovascular structures and diagnose complex anatomic disease. In most instances, cardiac anatomy is so well defined that cardiac catheterization is rarely necessary.

As echocardiography has evolved, the emphasis of a pediatric echocardiographic examination has shifted from an M-mode study yielding mostly functional information to a two-dimensional and color Doppler study yielding largely anatomic and physiologic information. Quantification of cardiovascular structure and function by echocardiography is not widely performed as many laboratories report the "most essential" (anatomic) information and forego the relatively time-consuming, labor intensive functional cardiac evaluation. This is particularly true in the pediatric laboratory in which ultrasound examinations often require extensive time and sedation to image complex congenital lesions. Accordingly, few pediatric echocardiography laboratories perform a quantitative examination. Automated quantification has not only improved efficiency, but it also has improved accuracy in laboratories.

Performing Acoustic Quantification in Children

Although the usually excellent image quality obtained in children facilitate endocardial tracking during an automatic border detection examination, there are issues unique to pediatric echocardiography that should be addressed in order to enhance quality. These are largely related with promoting patient cooperation and minimizing beat-to-beat variability of the data.

Optimizing Patient Cooperation

The cooperation of the pediatric patient is a prerequisite for any echocardiographic examination whether it involves M-mode, two-dimensional echocardiography or Doppler modalities. This is even more true for the case of echocardiographic examination using automated border techniques. Adjustments made to optimize endocardial tracking may be rendered useless by the slightest patient movement. Techniques for enhancing patient cooperation are similar to those used when performing a traditional echocardiographic examination. The newborn should be made comfortable by raising the room temperature, wrapping the legs and lower abdomen in warm blankets, using warm ultrasound gel, and providing further warmth with a radiant warmer. In addition, feeding of a baby can improve patient's comfort . The older child (3 - 18 year old), who is generally cooperative but may become restless, can be entertained with audiovisual media in the examining room.

Some children (particularly in the infant and toddler age groups) will not cooperate enough to perform an adequate examination. These patients require sedation (pentobarbital 3-5 mg/kg orally). When a child is sedated, she/he should be monitored appropriately (*i.e.* blood pressure, oximeter, and echocardiography itself).

Minimizing Beat-to-Beat Variability

Variability in on-line border detection measurements may be due to 1) patient movement, 2) respiratory-induced changes in image quality or 3) sonographer movement of the hand-held transducer. In the adult patient, the intraventricular volume is relatively large, so that the variations in measurements produced by these factors is relatively small. However, since volumes are smaller in children, the variability introduced by these factors may be more substantial. Reducing patient movement is best done by enhancing patient cooperation as described above. Sedation may be necessary.

The respiratory movement of the patient's chest can greatly influence endocardial tracking. In particular, inspiration may cause lung parenchyma to enter the echocardiographic field. Since this is a bright echo density, it is detected by the automatic border detection program producing marked attenuation of the ultrasonic signals resulting in significant change in the waveforms (Figure 8.1).

In adults, this problem is circumvented by having the patient hold her/his breath at end-expiration (when images are best and endocardial tracking is optimal). Children less than 13 to 15 year old cannot be expected to cooperate in this manner. Therefore, a respirometer is required to perform an accurate examination. The data obtained of at end-expiration is suitable for analysis. Alternatively, eliminating inaccurate information during inspiration can be facilitated by using signal averaging techniques with threshold values set at appropriate levels to filter all data except those occurring during end-expiration.

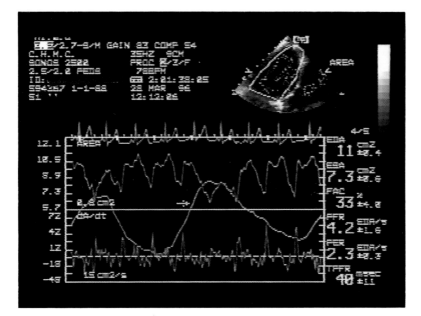

Figure 8.1. Left ventricular acoustic quantification waveforms in an eight-year-old boy from an apical 4-chamber view. The top waveform is the electrocardiogram. The second waveform is the area of the left ventricle as a function of time. The third waveform is the respirometer. The fourth waveform is the derivative of the area as a function of time. During inspiration (arrow) the left ventricular area waveform decreases in amplitude. Note that at end expiration the area waveform baseline is stable.

Endocardial tracking will be optimized by finding the best echocardiographic window and maintaining the image. Therefore, it is important for the transducer position to remain as steady as possible. In these cases, a two person approach may be necessary. Tracking can be enhanced by having the sonographer hold the transducer with both hands ensuring stability, while a second operator adjusts the echocardiographic system's settings.

Normal Pediatric Values

The normal values for left ventricular functional indexes obtained by automatic quantification in children between the ages of 6 weeks and 18 years are shown in Table 8.1 as obtained in our laboratory. A typical ventricular waveform is shown in Figure 8.2.

Table 8.1. Normal values for left ventricular indices in children.

	Short axis plane (mitral valve level)	Longitudinal plane (four-chamber)
Fractional area change (%)	52 - 70	21 - 38
Indexed peak filling rate* (s^{-1})	4.7 - 7.9	1.7 - 3.5
Indexed peak emptying rate* (s^{-1})	3.6 - 5.9	1.4 - 3.0

* Expressed in units of end-diastolic volume per second (the rates are normalized to the end-diastolic volume of the coresponding cardiac cycle).

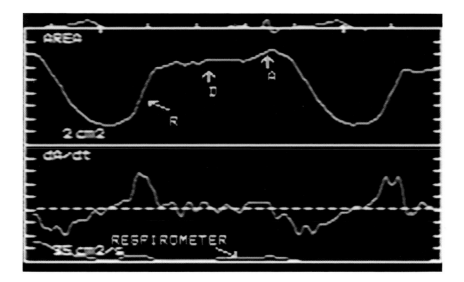

Figure 8.2. Left ventricular acoustic quantification waveforms obtained from a parasternal short axis view. The first waveform is the electrocardiogram. The second waveform is the area of the left ventricle as a function of time. The third waveform is the derivative of the area as a function of time. The fourth waveform is the respirometer. The three phases of ventricular filling (the rapid filling phase (R), diastasis (D), and atrial contraction (A) are delineated.

On-line analysis is not limited to the left ventricle. Indeed, any chamber or blood vessel can be evaluated. Assessment of left atrial size and function, for example, provides additional information regarding diastolic left ventricular function [1,2]. Normal values of left atrial functional indices for children are shown in Table 8.2. Obtaining accurate information on left atrial function can be difficult in children because the stability of left atrial waveforms are very sensitive to changes in respiration. Since most children cannot cooperate enough to suspend respiration, it is imperative that measurement of left atrial indices be obtained at end-expiration.

Table 8.2. Normal values of left atrial fractional indices in children.

Fractional area change in systole (%)	38 - 64
Indexed peak filling rate in systole* (s^{-1})	2.6 - 4.7
Indexed peak emptying rate in diastole* (s^{-1})	3.2 - 6.8

* Same as in Table 8.1.

The correlation of these functional indices with off-line analysis methods has been well established in the adult population. In children, too, there is excellent correlation between fractional area change assessed by automated quantification with that assessed by off-line methods. We have measured fractional area change by these two methods before, during and after dobutamine stress testing (Table 8.3). In all three conditions, an acceptable correlation between automatic quantification and off-line measurements was found. However, this correlation is slightly reduced at peak dobutamine infusion rates probably due to limited visualization of endocardium, which in turn compromises the endocardial tracking of the small left ventricular chamber area. As in adults, acoustic quantification excludes all portions of the mitral valve apparatus and trabeculi. Therefore, the blood pool cavity areas tend to be smaller and the function measurements tend to be higher with the on-line technique versus off-line analysis. This is also apparent in Table 8.3.

Table 8.3. Correlations of assessment of left ventricular fractional area change by acoustic quantification and by off-line methods at different inotropic states.

	On-line	Off-line	r	p
Rest	62 ± 14	53 ± 10	0.76	0.001
Maximum dobutamine	74 ± 19	67 ± 12	0.66	0.004
After dobutamine	58 ± 13	52 ± 12	0.76	0.001

On-line analysis consistently yielded significantly higher functional index measurements compared to off-line digitization. Therefore, the normal values for fractional area change are slightly higher than those reported for off-line methods (Table 8.1).

Review of Table 1 reveals significant differences between estimated left ventricular function in the short axis cardiac plane and left ventricular function in the cardiac longitudinal plane. Specifically, fractional area change and the left ventricular filling and emptying rates are greater in the short axis plane at the level of the mitral valve than corresponding indices measured in the longitudinal plane of the left ventricle. These findings confirm previous work using off-line measurements demonstrating that ejection fraction calculated from data in the short axis basal plane was consistently higher than ejection fraction incorporating longitudinal axis data [3]. These differences can be explained on the basis of two possible mechanisms. First, left ventricular function in the short axis cardiac plane may be lower at the apex than at the base [4]. Thus, an assessment of function from the short axis plane which incorporates data from base to apex may be expected to exhibit the expected variability. Regional pressure gradients within the left ventricular cavity have been identified and may explain regional differences in function. The characterization of these functional differences is controversial. Some studies show that the apical transverse plane has higher function than the basal transverse plane [5]. However, other investigators have shown that fractional area change is greater at the base than at the apex [6].

Developmental Changes

The ventricular area waveform obtained with acoustic quantification can delineate the three phases of diastole: rapid filling, diastasis, and atrial filling (Figure 8.3).

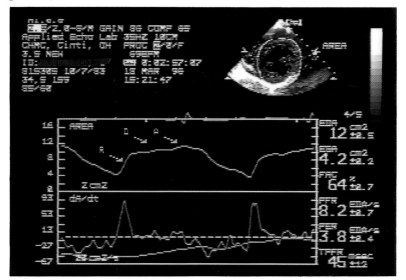

Figure 8.3. Left ventricular acoustic quantification waveforms from a parasternal short axis view in a 12-year-old girl. Ventricular filling is almost totally due to rapid filling (R). Diastasis (D) and atrial contraction (A) contribute very little to total ventricular filling.

The percent of total ventricular filling contributed by each of these phases can be measured. In normal adults the percent of total ventricular filling due to atrial contraction has been reported to be as high as 32% [7]. These findings have been recently corroborated in adults employing Doppler techniques demonstrating less prominent passive ventricular filling with increasing age coupled with augmented atrial contraction contribution [2, 8-10]. Increasing dependence on atrial contraction for ventricular filling with age has been attributed to increased myocardial stiffness with age. Not surprisingly, therefore, filling of the relatively compliant left ventricle of children would be almost exclusively dependent on passive filling with minimal atrial contribution. Indeed, in children, atrial contraction accounts for only 20% of total LV filling (Table 8.4, Figure 8.3). Compared to Chenzbraun's data obtained in adults, passive left ventricular filling (*i.e.* rapid filling and diastasis) is more prominent in the pediatric age group. On the other hand, in neonates, ventricular compliance is reduced [11] suggesting that atrial contraction may play, as in the elderly, a more important role.

Table 8.4. Percent of total diastolic filling contributed by rapid filling, diastasis and atrial contraction in children.

% total diastolic filling contributed by:	Short axis plane (mitral valve level)	Longitudinal plane
Rapid filling	66 - 80	64 - 76
Diastasis	7 - 20	12 - 21
Atrial contraction	6 - 20	9 - 19

Attributing these findings solely to changes in ventricular compliance may be an oversimplification. The mechanisms governing early ventricular filling are complex and dictated by 1) the diastolic atrio-ventricular pressure gradient, 2) the rate of left ventricular isovolumic pressure fall, 3) the left atrial pressure at the time of mitral valve opening, 4) the left ventricular end-systolic volume 5) and myocardial stiffness. The atrial contribution to filling correlates with the length of the atrial fibers prior to be initiation of contraction such that less passive ventricular filling will result in increased atrial fiber stretch and augmented atrial contraction. All of above mentioned mechanisms need to be accounted when filling patterns are interpreted in the newborn.

Measuring Function in Ventricles of Unusual Geometry

Pediatric echocardiographers are often asked to assess the ventricular function of chambers with peculiar geometric configurations. For example, determination of right ventricular function is particularly important in patients undergoing Mustard or Senning operations for transposition of the great vessels. In these patients, the right ventricle assumes the role of the systemic ventricle. In adolescence, almost 50% of such patients will experience heart failure. There are also many other congenital anomalies that are associated with unusual ventricular configurations. Tricuspid atresia and the hypoplastic left heart syndrome are lesions that exhibit unusual ventricular geometry associated with univentricular heart physiology as part of their pathophysiologic manifestations.

The quantification and serial assessment of ventricular function in these patients is difficult. Often, the clinician has no quantitative estimate of ventricular function at all. In all these conditions, the "ice-pick" view provided by the traditional measurement M-Mode derived function (fractional shortening) is inaccurate, providing very little information about global ventricular performance. Measurement of fractional area change off-line by two-dimensional echocardiography is often inaccurate because identification of endocardial boundaries off-line is difficult.

Functional assessment of these ventricles can be evaluated by using on-line analysis. On-line quantification is valuable in assessing and serially measuring ventricular function in these patients as it is performed at the time of the study allowing for easier identification of endocardium than is possible off-line from videotaped images [12]. In addition, on-line quantification provides a better global functional measurement of the univentricular heart.

The assessment of ventricular function in the hypoplastic left heart syndrome is particularly important. The reduced number of infant heart donors for transplantation and the improvement in survival rates with surgical palliation have made this a more attractive treatment option. Because morbidity during the 3 palliative stages (Norwood procedure, bi-directional Glenn, Fontan completion) is related to the degree of dysfunction of the single right ventricle, serial assessment of ventricular performance is crucial.

Using on-line quantification, the function of the systemic right ventricle in patients with hypoplastic left heart syndrome can now be studied (Figure 8.4).

Interestingly, this ventricle exhibits significantly depressed function compared to that of normal patients (Table 8.5). Depressed systolic function is indicated by the reduced fractional area change and peak emptying rate. This may be related to an intrinsic myocardial dysfunction linked to the bypass surgical procedure, inadequate hypertrophy, or endomyocardial fibroelastosis. Alternatively, systolic dysfunction may result from the ventricle being deprived of adequate ventricular interaction. Fogel *et al.* [13] have demonstrated that myocardial strain is markedly different in univentricular hearts such as a systemic right ventricle (*e.g.* hypoplastic left heart syndrome) compared to a ventricle that is part of a dual chamber circulation (*e.g.* transposition of the great vessels with atrial inversion operation).

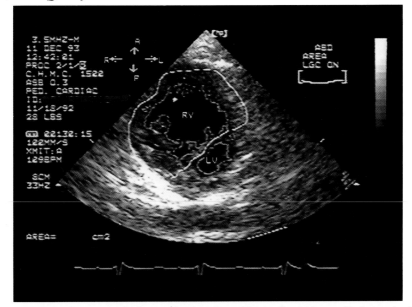

Figure 8.4. Parasternal short axis view in a 13-month-old boy with hypoplastic left heart syndrome. Endocardial tracking (orange line) is demonstrated on the compensatorily enlarged systemic right ventricle (RV) and the hypoplastic left ventricle (LV). The region of interest (white line) is drawn around the right ventricle. A-anterior, L-left, P-posterior, R-right.

Table 8.5. Systemic right ventricular function in children with hypoplastic left heart syndrome. FAC - area change, PFR - peak filling rate, PER - peak emptying rate. * same as in Table 8.1

	AFTER			**NORMALS**
	Stage I	Stage II	Stage III	
SYSTOLIC				
Short axis - atrial FAC (%)	39±2	42±4	35±8	61±10
Apical - ventricular fractional FAC (%)	34±6	31±6	29±5	31±11
Short axis - ventricular PER* (s^{-1})	3.1±0.3	3.9±0.7	3.4±1.3	5.3±1.3
Apical - ventricular PER* (s^{-1})	2.3±0.4	2.6±0.4	2.2±0.2	2.4±0.9
DIASTOLIC				
Short axis - ventricular PFR* (s^{-1})	3.9±0.2	5.9±0.7	3.1±0.5	6.6±2.3
Apical - ventricular PFR* (s^{-1})	2.8±0.7	3.7±1.0	2.6±0.7	3.2±1.2
Left or right atrial fractional FAC (%)	37±17	31±13	48±15	55±16
Rapid filling contribution (%)	63±20	60±11	76±9	73±5
Diastasis contribution (%)	26±14	15±11	7±9	16±6
Atrial contraction contribution (%)	11±6	25±5	17±5	12±4

On-line quantification data indicate that patients with hypoplastic left heart syndrome also exhibit diastolic dysfunction. Peak filling rate is depressed indicative of abnormalities in passive filling. In addition, the atrial contribution to ventricular filling becomes more important as the patients are converted to the physiology conferred by the Fontan operation (Figure 8.5). A possible explanation for this conversion has been suggested by Gewillig *et al.* [14]. These investigators placed systemic to pulmonary arterial shunts surgically (to simulate volume overload in the palliated state of the univentricular circulation) in dogs and studied their ventricular filling patterns. After the chronic volume overload was removed, rapid filling was blunted. Since this finding was associated with an increased ventricular mass-to-volume ratio, the authors concluded that diastolic filling is impaired after relief of volume overload because of increased viscosity of blood and inertia of the myocardium.

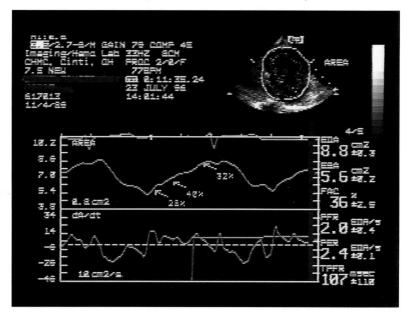

Figure 8.5. Acoustic quantification waveforms of the systemic right ventricle in a 6-year-old girl that has undergone all three stages of the Norwood procedure. The rapid filling phase contributes only 28% to total left ventricular filling. Diastasis contributes 40%, and atrial contraction contributes 32% to total systemic ventricular filling. These results suggest altered compliance of the systemic right ventricle. The peak filling rate $(2.0s^{-1})$ is decreased.

As experience with on-line quantification in accumulated, it will be important to study these issues in other clinical conditions associated with unusual ventricular geometry. For example, this technique can be utilized to determine if single systemic right ventricles (*e.g.* in hypoplastic left heart) perform similarly to single systemic left ventricles (*e.g.* in tricuspid atresia). It can also be employed to elucidate if a systemic single right ventricle performs similarly to a systemic right ventricle that is part of a dual circulation (*e.g.* in patients with an atrial baffle for the arterial switch operation). Results of such studies may help clinicians recognize ventricular dysfunction more accurately and dictate medical treatment and surgical referrals more appropriately.

Detecting Diastolic Dysfunction

Although Doppler indices of diastolic ventricular function are extremely useful, they also have significant limitations. These indices are not only dependent on the diastolic properties of the ventricle, but also depend on afterload, preload, aging, and heart rate [15]. Therefore, assessment of diastolic function remains difficult [16]. Since the effect of heart rate on these indices is probably the single prevailing limiting factor in the pediatric population, a diastolic index which is not dependent on heart rate would be valuable. Preliminary work suggests that peak ventricular filling rate obtained from on-line border detection is very sensitive for detection of diastolic dysfunction and, at the same time, is heart rate independent [17] (see Chapter 5).

Although peak filling rate has traditionally been measured by M-mode echocardiography, its measurement by on-line acoustic quantification methods is more accurate. M-mode-derived peak filling rate evaluates LV filling rate in a single location of the left ventricle. On-line acoustic quantification-derived peak filling rate confers a global assessment of ventricular filling obtained from the two-dimensional section of the left ventricle. Indeed, in a population of children with documented diastolic dysfunction, peak filling rate by on-line border detection successfully detected disease in 90% of the cases whereas peak filling rate by M-mode echocardiography detected disease in only 20% of the patients. Not surprisingly, on-line acoustic quantification peak filling rates were more sensitive than Doppler indices (*e.g.* E/A ratio was able to detect disease in only 50% of the patients) [17].

Similar to the Doppler spectral pattern of the mitral inflow velocity, the ventricular diastolic waveform obtained on-line reflects the left ventricular-left atrial pressure gradient. It is, therefore, valuable in detecting the two main types of diastolic abnormalities: impaired relaxation and restrictive physiology. Abnormal ventricular relaxation lengthens the isovolumic relaxation time and the mitral deceleration time, and shifts the preponderance of ventricular filling to the atrial contraction phase of diastole. Restrictive ventricular physiology, on the other hand, results in more rapid equilibration of the left atrial and left ventricular pressures in early to mid-diastole, thus shortening the mitral deceleration time. Under these conditions the left atrium largely serves as a conduit for ventricular filling, the majority of which occurs during early diastole. By the time atrial contraction occurs, the left ventricular pressure has risen to such a degree that the pressure generated from atrial contraction cannot overcome the left ventricular pressure resulting in minimal filling during mid and late diastole.

The percentages of total left ventricular filling contributed by rapid filling, diastasis, and atrial contraction are, therefore, useful indexes to detect diastolic dysfunction. In the pediatric population, the majority of left ventricular filling normally occurs during rapid filling in early diastole. Diastolic dysfunction can be manifested by a reduction of rapid filling and/or an augmentation of LV filling due to atrial contraction or diastasis. For example, children with congenital aortic stenosis exhibit a progressive decrease in the percent of rapid filling and progressive increase in the degree of filling occurring during both atrial contraction and diastasis. (Figure 8.6) These results are consistent with previous studies conducted with M-mode echocardiography [18] or venticulography [19] that demonstrate depressed early diastolic filling in patients with aortic stenosis. These diastolic functional abnormalities correlate best with decreasing aortic valve area and increasing pressure gradient. Therefore, they may be secondary to coronary artery perfusion abnormalities rather than degree of ventricular hypertrophy.

Left ventricular filling patterns can also be useful in detecting diastolic dysfunction in children with systemic metabolic diseases. In young patients with insulin-dependent diabetes mellitus, for example, the percent filling due to atrial contraction is increased and that due to rapid filling is reduced (Figure 8.7). Since global left ventricular systolic function is preserved in these patients, the presence of these ventricular filling abnormalities may aid in the earlier detection of myocardial involvement in diabetic patients.

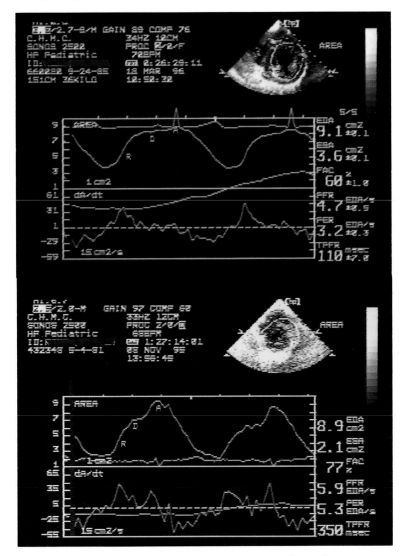

Figure 8.6. Left ventricular acoustic quantification waveforms from a parasternal short axis view in a 10-year-old boy with mild (22 mmHg) aortic stenosis (Top) and in a 14-year-old girl with moderate (53 mmHg) aortic stenosis (Bottom). The left ventricular filling patterns in the patient with mild aortic stenosis are normal. However, the filling patterns in the patient with moderate aortic stenosis are distinctly abnormal with accentuated filling due to atrial contraction and relatively less filling due to rapid filling.

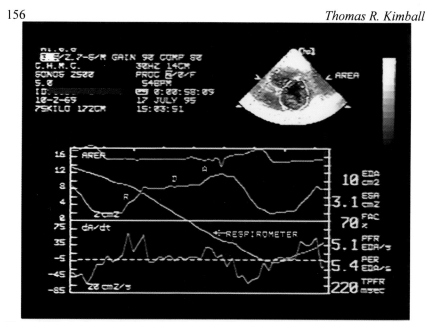

Figure 8.7. Left ventricular acoustic quantification waveforms from a parasternal short axis view in a 25-year-old male with insulin-dependent diabetes mellitus. Even with a relatively short duration of diabetes (17 years), this patient exhibits abnormal left ventricular filling with accentuation of the atrial component (A) and decreased filling during the rapid filling phase (R). D-diastasis.

Markers for Transplant Rejection

Timely diagnosis of acute cardiac allograft rejection is critical for the survival of heart transplant patients. The mainstay of diagnosis remains the use of endomyocardial biopsy. However, in children the risks of biopsy and the difficulty of obtaining repeated central venous access make this procedure a less desirable diagnostic option. Therefore, investigators have employed echocardiographic parameters to determine their sensitivity in diagnosing allograft rejection. In adult patients, various measurements including LV mass, left ventricular fractional shortening and wall thickening, left ventricular compliance and transmitral inflow velocities have been studied, but none of these indexes has resulted in a reliable indicator of allograft rejection [20, 21]. In children, Doppler indices are less useful because of higher resting heart rates compared to adults [22]. Even pediatric studies employing M-mode and two-dimensional indices have shown conflicting results [23-25]; therefore the echocardiographic diagnosis of allograft rejection in children remains elusive.

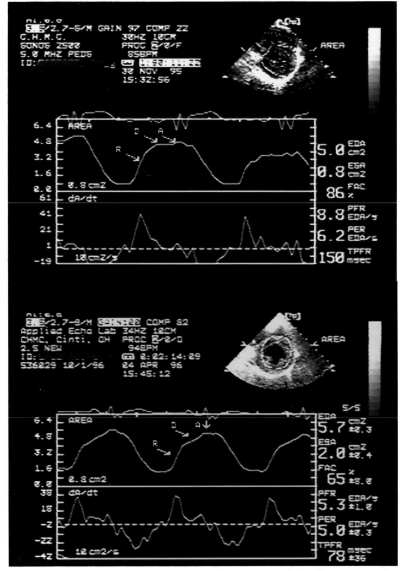

Figure 8.8. Left ventricular acoustic quantification waveforms from a parasternal short axis view in an 8-year-old girl with an orthotopic heart transplant before rejection (A) and during an episode of biopsy-proven ISHLT grade 2 rejection (B). Before rejection, the ventricular filling patterns are normal. During rejection, there is a diminution in the filling occurring during the rapid filling phase (R) and an accentuation of the filling during diastasis (D). A - atrial contraction.

On-line quantification indices may, however, become valuable in the diagnosis of rejection. Since these parameters evaluate ventricular performance in ways that have previously not been possible, and since they may be more accurate in the assessment of more subtle disease, these indices may be able to detect earlier alterations changes in function that occur during acute rejection. Preliminary data suggest that analysis of left ventricular filling patterns may be valuable in detecting rejection. Specifically, data suggest that the percentage of left ventricular filling during the rapid filling phase may be attenuated during rejection (Figure 8.8). If these findings can be validated in a prospective study, left ventricular filling patterns may become a noninvasive reference standard for the diagnosis of allograft rejection in children.

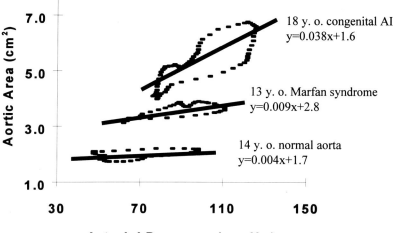

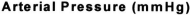

Figure 8.9. Pressure area loops of the ascending aorta derived from simultaneous acoustic quantification area waveforms and indirect carotid pulse trace. Loops from three patient are shown. The regression line for each of the three loops is also demonstrated. The slope of each regression line is the aortic compliance for each patient. A normal pressure area loop from a 14-year-old girl is shown at the bottom. Compliance is 0.004 cm²/mmHg. The middle pressure area loop is from a 13-year-old boy with Marfan's syndrome. The compliance of his aorta is more than double that of the patient with a normal aorta. Finally, the top pressure area loop is from an 18-year-old girl with congenital aortic insufficiency. The aortic compliance of her ascending aorta is almost 10 times normal.

Assessment of Physiologic Performance and Systemic Arterial Function

The assessment of ventriculo-arterial coupling has become important as investigators have realized that the arterial system is not merely a conduit for blood but also a capacitance vessel that modifies cardiac flow from pulsatile to continuous in order to exchange metabolites effectively. Therefore, regional elastic properties of the aorta have been measured in adults to quantify the capacitance of the systemic arterial system [26] (see Chapter 6). Investigators have used on-line quantification techniques of images of the thoracic aorta obtained with transesophageal echocardiography and indirect subclavian arterial pulse tracings to generate pressure-area loops. From these loops indices directly proportional to regional aortic compliance can be derived. The same technique can be applied to children. Preliminary data show that aortic compliance is altered in certain pediatric cardiovascular diseases (Figure 8.9). These measures of compliance will be helpful in providing insight into mechanisms of vascular disease in children with congenital heart disease.

Conclusion

On-line quantification of cardiovascular function is a new and particularly exciting technique in pediatrics. These measurements allow assessment of ventricular and arterial function in ways never possible heretofore. A more global assessment of ventricular performance is provided relatively quick and easy. The superior image quality usually obtained in children as compared to adults, combined with the improvement in accuracy of measurements make on-line quantification techniques important new modalities in the assessment of pediatric cardiovascular disease.

References

1. Clarkson PBM, Wheeldon NM, Lim PO, Pringle SD, MacDonald TM: Left atrial size and function: Assessment using echocardiographic automatic boundary detection. *Br Heart J* 1995;74:664-670.
2. Triposkiadis F, Tentolouris K, Androulakis A, Trikas A, Toutouzas K, Kyriakidis M, Gialafos J, Toutouzas P: Left atrial mechanical function in the healthy elderly: new insights from a combined assessment of changes in atrial volume and transmitral flow velocity. *J Am Soc Echocardiogr* 1995;8:801-809.
3. Fast J, Jacobs S: Limits of reproducibility of cross-sectional echocardiographic measurement of left ventricular ejection fraction. *Int J Cardiol* 1990;28:67-72.

4. Gorcsan J, Lazar JM, Schulman DS, Follansbee WP: Comparison of left ventricular function by echocardiographic automated border detection and by radionuclide ejection fraction. *Am J Cardiol* 1993:72:810-815.

5. Pearlman JD, Triulzi MO, King ME, Newell J, Weyman AE: Limits of normal left ventricular dimensions in growth and development: analysis of dimensions and variance in the two-dimensional echocardiograms of 268 normal healthy subjects. *J Am Coll Cardiol* 1988;12:1432-1441.

6. Assman PE, Slager CJ, van der Borden SG, Sutherland GR, Roelandt JR: Reference systems in echocardiographic quantitative wall motion analysis with registration of respiration. *J Am Soc Echo* 1991;4:224-234.

7. Chenzbraun A, Pinto FJ, Popylisen S, Schnittger I, Popp RL: Filling patterns in left ventricular hypertrophy: a combined acoustic quantification and Doppler study. *J Am Coll Cardiol* 1994;23:1179-1185.

8. Sartori MP, Quinoes MA, Kuo LC: Relation of Doppler-derived left ventricular filling parameters to age and radius/thickness ratio in normal and pathologic states. *Am J Cardiol* 1987; 59:1179-1182.

9. Miyatake K, Okamoto M, Kinoshita N, Owa M, Nakasone I, Sakakibara H, Nimura Y: Augmentation of atrial contribution to left ventricular inflow with aging as assessed by intracardiac Doppler flowmetry. *Am J Cardiol* 1984;53:586-589.

10. Byrg RJ, Williams GA, Labovitz AJ: Effect of aging on left ventricular diastolic filling in normal subjects. *Am J Cardiol* 1987;59:971-974.

11. Romero T, Covell J, Friedman WF: A comparison of pressure-volume relations of the fetal, newborn, and adult heart. *Am J Physiol* 1972; 222:1285-1292.

12. Kimball TR, Witt SA, Khoury PR, Daniels SR: Automated echocardiographic analysis of systemic ventricular performance in hypoplastic left heart syndrome. *J Am Soc Echocardiogr* 1996; 9:629-636.

13. Fogel MA, Weinberg PM, Fellows KE, Hoffman EA: A study in ventricular-ventricular interaction. Single right ventricles compared with systemic right ventricles in a dual-chamber circulation. *Circulation* 1995; 92:219-230.

14. Gewillig M, Daenen W, Aubert A, Van der Hauwaert L: Abolishment of chronic volume overload. Implications for diastolic function of the systemic ventricle immediately after Fontan repair. *Circulation* 1991; 86 (suppl II):II-93-II-99.

15. Benjamin EJ, Levy D, Anderson FM, Wolf PA, Plehn JF, Evans JC, Comai K, Fuller DL, St. John Sutton M: Determinants of Doppler indices of left ventricular diastolic function in normal subjects (The Framingham Heart study). *Am J Cardiol* 1992; 70:508-515.

16. Shapiro SM Bersohn MM, Laks MM: In search of the holy grail: the study of diastolic ventricular function by the use of echocardiography. *J Am Coll Cardiol* 1991; 17:1517-1519.

17. Kimball TR, Witt SA, Daniels SR, Khoury PR, Meyer RA: The role of automatic endocardial edge detection in the evaluation of left ventricular diastolic function in children. *J Am Soc Echocardiogr* 1996; 9:18-26.

18. Fifer MA, Borow KM, Colan SD, Lorell KH: Early diastolic left ventricular function in children and adults with aortic stenosis. *J Am Coll Cardiol* 1985; 5:1147-1154.

19. Murakami T, Hess OM, Gage JE, Grimm J, Krayenbuehl HP: Diastolic filling dynamics in patients with aortic stenosis. *Circulation* 1986; 73:1162-1174.
20. Valantine HA, Fowler MB, Hunt SA, Naasz C, Hatle LK, Billingham ME, Stinson,EB, Popp R: Changes in Doppler echocardiographic indexes of left ventricular function as potential markers of acute cardiac rejection. *Circulation* 1987; 76(Suppl):V86-V92.
21. Mannaerts H, Balk A, Simoons M, Tijssen J, van der Borden SG, Zondervan P, Sutherland G, Roelandt JRTC: Changes in left ventricular function and wall thickness in heart transplant recipients and their relation to acute rejection: an assessment by digitised M mode echocardiography. *Br Heart J* 1992; 68:356-364.
22. Riggs TW, Snider AR: Respiratory influence on right and left ventrcular diastolic function in normal children. *Am J Cardiol* 1989; 63:858-861.
23. Boucek MM, Mathis CM, Boucek RJ, Hodgkin DP, Kanakrajeh MS, McCormack J, Gundry SR, Bailey LL: Prospective evaluation of echocardiography for primary rejection surveillance after infant heart transplantation: comparison with endomyocardial biopsy. *J Heart Lung Transplant* 1994; 13:66-73.
24. Zales VR, Crawford S, Backer CL, Pahl E, Webb CL, Lynch P, Mavroudis C, Benson DW: Role of endomyocardial biopsy in rejection surveillance after heart transplantation in neonates and children. *J Am Coll Cardiol* 1994; 23:766-771.
25. Kimball TR, Witt AS, Daniels SR, Khoury PR, Meyer RA: Frequency and significance of left ventricular thickening in transplanted hearts in children. *Am J Cardiol* 1996; 77:77-80.
26. Lang RM, Cholley BP, Korcarz C, Marcus RH, Shroff SG: Measurement of regional elastic properites of the human aorta. A new application of transesophageal echocardiography with automated border detection and calibrated subcavian pulse tracings. *Circulation* 1994; 90:1875-1882.

9 Quantitative Intraoperative Echocardiographic Assessment of Ventricular Function

John Gorcsan III

Transesophageal echocardiography has become an important tool in the operating room to assist in the management of patients undergoing cardiovascular procedures. In addition to immediately evaluating the results of valvular surgery, transesophageal echocardiographic imaging has made an impact in optimizing intraoperative therapy through the assessment of left ventricular filling, regional wall motion, and global cardiac function [1-4]. Echocardiograhic automated border detection which uses ultrasound backscatter analysis is well suited to the transesophageal approach because of the high resolution imaging and favorable signal-to-noise ratios obtained. This discussion will review the validation studies in animal models and in humans for assessing ventricular volume by echocardiographic automated border detection and focus on its application for the quantitative assessment of left ventricular function in the operating room.

Cross Sectional Area To Assess Changes In Left Ventricular Volume

The automated border detection system uses backscatter data to differentiate between tissue and blood ultrasound densities for each pixel along each scan line within the ultrasound sector [5,6]. Left ventricular cavity area is then calculated within a user-defined region of interest in real time. Because echocardiographic data constructed on-line are two-dimensional, the relationship between left ventricular cross-sectional area and true volume must be first carefully considered. This relationship was studied in our laboratory in an isolated canine heart preparation where an intraventricular balloon was placed to directly control and measure true left ventricular volume [7]. The isovolumically contracting heart was placed in an *ex-vivo* apparatus with the echocardiography transducer in epicardial contact at the mid-ventricular short-axis plane for simultaneous automated border detection measures of area during gradual step-wise changes in volume of the balloon. A linear relationship of changes in area to changes in true volume was observed in a series of seven hearts, with a group mean r=0.97±0.02, and mean SEE=0.31±0.08 cm² (Figure 9.1). This relationship was linear within the physiological range of values, but became curvilinear at low ventricular volumes. In addition, the deformational changes of the left ventricle as it became more spherical during isovolumic contraction were minimal (<0.4 cm²) in 6 of 7 dogs but a cycle specific change of 28% was observed in 1 dog.

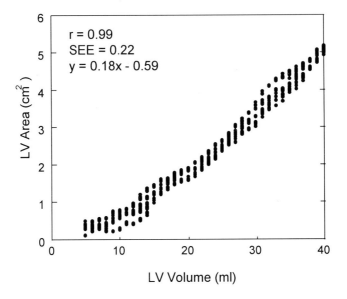

Figure 9.1. Plot of an example of the relationship of cross-sectional area by automated border detection with true volume in an isolated canine heart preparation. Reprinted with permission from the *J Am Soc Echocardiogr* 1993;6:482-489.

On-line changes in left ventricular cross-sectional area were also compared with changes in stroke volume determined by an electromagnetic flow probe placed on the ascending aorta in an open-chest canine model with intact circulation [8]. Left ventricular filling and ejection were rapidly altered by repeated inferior vena caval occlusions (Figure 9.2).

INFERIOR VENA CAVAL OCCLUSION

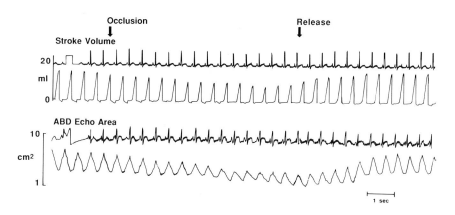

Figure 9.2. An example of simultaneous changes in echocardiographic automated border detection (ABD) area at midventricular short-axis plane and stroke volume by an electromagnetic flow probe during inferior vena caval occlusion from an open-chest dog model. Reprinted with permission from the *Am Heart J* 1993; 125:1316-1323.

Simultaneous changes in stroke area (end-diastolic area - end-systolic area) by echocardiographic automated border detection were consistently correlated with changes in stroke volume (Figure 9.3). These studies have demonstrated a relationship between changes in left ventricular cross-sectional area and changes in volume which is predictably linear within physiologic ranges. These data support the previous findings of other investigators who have demonstrated the ability of two-dimensions to accurately track changes in true volume assessed by sonomicrometry in a canine model during multiple hemodynamic alterations including transient occlusions of the inferior vena cava, aorta, and pulmonary artery, and hypovolemia induced by phlebotomy [9].

Transesophageal echocardiographic imaging of the mid-ventricular short-axis plane from the transgastric window has been useful in the operating room to monitor changes in regional left ventricular function and to estimate left ventricular volume [2-4,10]. Although there is no accurate formula to calculate absolute volume from this plane, changes in cross-sectional area have also been shown to reliably follow changes in left ventricular volume and function [11]. Cheung *et al.* has shown that off-line measures of left ventricular end-diastolic area using intraoperative transesophageal echocardiography were sensitive to changes in preload induced by blood loss of as little as 2.5% of the patients estimated blood volume [12]. These changes in end-diastolic area were observed in a group of 30 patients including patients with normal left ventricular function as well as patients with regional dysfunction. On-line recordings of left ventricular cross-sectional area using automated border detection have also been shown to track changes in stroke volume in patients undergoing coronary artery bypass surgery (Figure 9.4) [13].

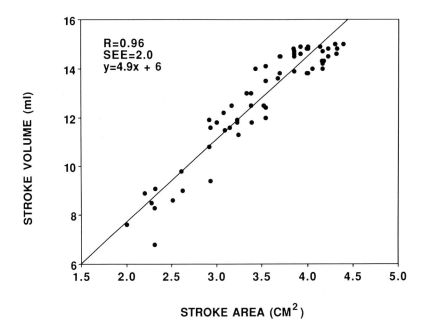

Figure 9.3. An example of changes in stroke volume vs. stroke area (end-diastolic area - end-systolic area) during inferior vena caval occlusion from a dog model. Reprinted with permission from the *Am Heart J* 1993; 125:1316-1323.

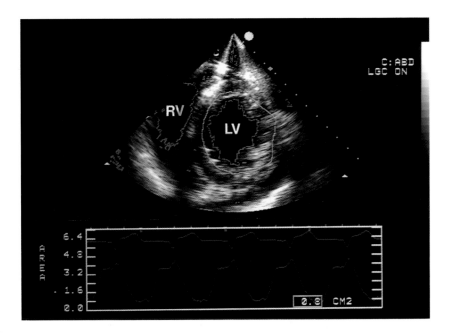

Figure 9.4. Transesophageal echocardiographic image at midventricular short-axis plane demonstrating automated border detection measures of left ventricular (LV) cavity area. RV; right ventricle. Reprinted with permission from the *Am J Cardiol*, 1993;72:721-727.

In a series of nine patients, we obtained simultaneous recordings of mid-ventricular cross-sectional area using transesophageal echocardiographic automated border detection and ventricular ejection volume using an aortic electromagnetic flow probe were acquired during changes induced by inferior vena caval occlusions (Figure 9.5). A close linear relationship between changes in stroke area (the difference of end-diastolic area and end-systolic area) and changes in stroke volume was observed with group mean r=0.94±0.03, SEE=0.33±0.12 cm² before cardiopulmonary bypass (n=8), and r=0.92±0.05, SEE=0.59±0.81 cm² after bypass (n=5). Five of these patients had regional wall motion abnormalities from coronary artery disease, and the mid-ventricular short-axis tomographic plane appeared to predict alterations in volume even in patients with regional dysfunction. However, it should be noted that the mean ejection fraction of this group of patients studied was 54±12%, indicating that the degree of left ventricular dysfunction was mild. It is uncertain if a similar close linear relationship between area and volume may exist in ventricles with more significant wall motion abnormalities, such as ventricular aneurysms [14]. Monitoring changes in cross-sectional area, however, does appear well suited to serially assess changes in left ventricular volume in individuals over time.

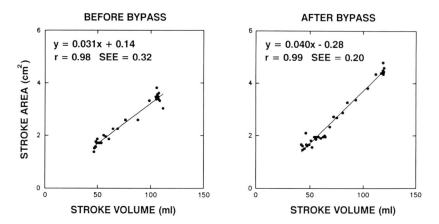

Figure 9.5. Examples of the linear relationship of changes in stroke volume with changes in stroke area (end-diastolic area - end-systolic area) during intraoperative inferior vena caval occlusion from a patient before and immediately after coronary artery bypass surgery. Reprinted with permission from the *Am J Cardiol*, 1993;72:721-727.

Automated Estimation of Left Ventricular Volume

Several investigators have previously validated the use of conventional single plane and biplane transesophageal echocardiography for determining left ventricular volumes and calculating ejection fractions from long axis tomographic planes. These approaches have included application of a modified Simpson's rule or area-length formulas to the transverse four-chamber or longitudinal two-chamber views. Smith *et al.* demonstrated a good correlation of single plane left ventricular end-diastolic volumes, end-systolic volumes, and ejection fraction with cineventriculography as a standard of reference using manual tracing of the endocardial borders (r=0.80-0.95) [15]. Hozumi *et al.* reported results with biplane transesophageal images which were comparable with left ventricular volumes calculated from similar transthoracic images in the same patients [16]. These studies, however, have suggested that these transesophageal views may underestimate ventricular volumes, in particular from the four-chamber view because of incomplete imaging of the LV apex.

Automated border detection algorithms have been developed to estimate volume from long axis images on-line (Hewlett-Packard, Andover, MA). These algorithms utilize either an automated area-length formula: $(8 \text{ area}^2)/ (3\pi \text{ length})$, or Simpson's rule which calculates volume from 20 equally spaced circular discs [17-19]. Morrissey *et al.* showed a significant linear relationship of echocardiographic automated border detection measures of volume with true volume measured by an intraventricular balloon in an ejecting canine model [17]. These automated volume algorithms have also been evaluated using the transesophageal approach (Figures 9.6A, 9.6B).

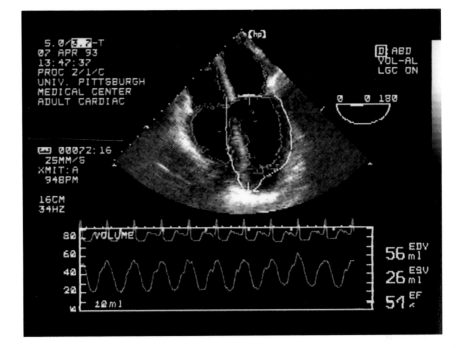

Figure 9.6(A): An example of transesophageal echocardiographic automated border detection from the transverse four-chamber plane with left ventricular volume estimated on-line by the area-length method. Reprinted with permission from the *Am Heart J* 1994;128:389-396.

The prototype transesophageal echocardiographic automated border detection volume software was evaluated in our laboratory in a closed-chest canine model where simultaneous volume was measured by a conductance catheter [19]. This multielectrode left ventricular catheter has been validated to track changes in volume on-line by determining alterations in blood conductivity [20,21]. Seven anesthetized dogs had simultaneous automated border detection volume using the Simpson's rule algorithm and conductance catheter volume recorded during steady state and during alterations induced by inferior vena caval balloon occlusions. Changes in relative volume by transesophageal automated border detection throughout the cardiac cycle were consistently related to steady state volume assessed by the conductance catheter; $r=0.93\pm0.03$, SEE=$10\pm2\%$ (Figure 9.7).

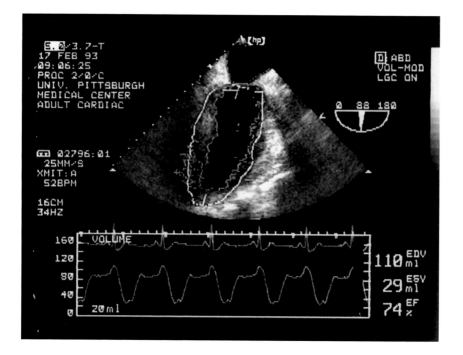

Figure 9.6(B). An example of transesophageal echocardiographic automated border detection from the longitudinal two-chamber plane with left ventricular volume estimated by the modified Simpson's rule. Reprinted with permission from the *Am Heart J* 1994;128:389-396.

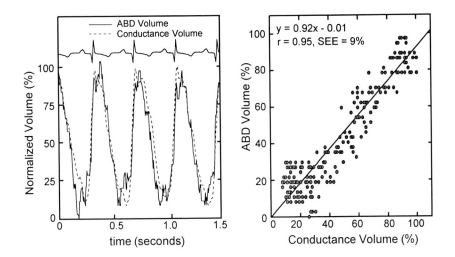

Figure 9.7. Left: Simultaneous steady-state transesophageal automated border detection (ABD) volume by Simpson's rule and conductance catheter volume from a canine model expressed as % to show similar relative changes throughout the cardiac cycle. Right: Linear regression plot of corresponding % ABD vs. % conductance volume. Reprinted with permission of the *Am Heart J* 1996;131:544-552.

When absolute steady state volume values were pooled and assessed by Bland-Altman analysis, an overall bias of -15 ml for automated echocardiographic measures was observed when compared with values obtained by the conductance catheter [22]. The respective relationships of end-diastolic volume and end-systolic volume by the two methods during alterations in preload were also highly linearly related. Close correlations were observed for end-diastolic volume (r=0.93±0.04) and end-systolic volume (r=0.89±0.04). However, end-diastolic volume and end-systolic volume values were less by the automated border detection with an overall bias of -10 ml and -8 ml, respectively. Differences in respective volume values appeared greatest with larger ventricular volumes.

Biplane transesophageal echocardiographic automated border detection has been used to estimate left ventricular stroke volume and cardiac output in humans undergoing cardiac surgery [18]. We compared simultaneous transesophageal automated border detection and thermodilution measures of cardiac output in 18 patients before and immediately after cardiopulmonary bypass. Automated volume measurements were independently assessed from the four-chamber view and the two-chamber. Both area-length and Simpson's rule formulas were tested. Technically satisfactory data were available in 22 of 33 studies (67%) from the four-chamber view, and 27 of 33 studies (82%) from the two-chamber view. The results of transesophageal echocardiographic automated border detection estimates of cardiac output correlated with thermodilution cardiac output are summarized in Figure 9.8. The area-length and Simpson's rule volume calculations were similar. Although significant correlations were consistently demonstrated, the four-chamber view tended to underestimate cardiac output, with a bias of -1.9 L/min. The degree of underestimation from the two-chamber view was less. These data demonstrate that cardiac output calculations by transesophageal echocardiographic automated border detection are feasible and accurate at detecting changes on-line. The observed bias with the prototype automated echocardiographic system is to slightly underestimate absolute values of cardiac output.

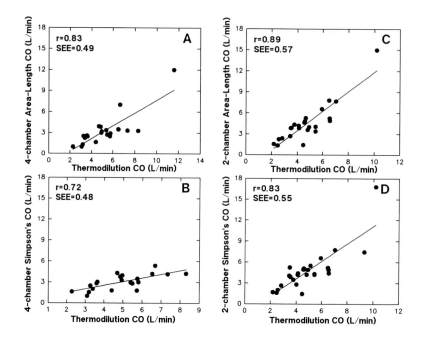

Figure 9.8. Results of the correlations of cardiac output (CO) from transesophageal automated border detection with simultaneous thermodilution CO. Reprinted with permission from the *Am Heart J* 1994;128:389-396.

Pressure-Volume and Pressure-Area Relations

The evaluation of left ventricular contraction with the pressure-volume diagram, as developed by Suga and Sagawa, has aided in our understanding of the fundamental mechanics of cardiac contractility, myocardial energetics, and coupling of pump function with the vasculature [23-25]. Pressure-volume relations have been an important means to determine left ventricular contractility because of their relative insensitivity to loading conditions. The linear slope of the end-systolic pressure-volume relationship examined over a wide range of values, as originally demonstrated in an isolated ejecting canine heart, can describe global left ventricular contractility (Figure 9.9). Although pressure-volume relations are not entirely insensitive to load in intact cardiovascular systems and are influenced by the autonomic nervous system, they have been an accepted standard to describe ventricular performance. The assessment of pressure-volume relations has been limited clinically by difficulties in acquiring on-line volume data, although measurement of ventricular pressure may be quite routine. The use of automated border detection with either cross-sectional area as a surrogate for left ventricular volume, or the automated volume algorithm has enabled the application of pressure-volume relations to clinical settings not possible previously, such as the operating room. Measures of ventricular contractility may be applied to a family of pressure-volume or pressure-area loops recorded over a range of different pressure and volume values. This is most commonly accomplished in a clinical or experimental setting by transiently occluding inferior vena caval inflow with a balloon occluder to rapidly decrease left ventricular pressure and volume. This method to rapidly alter preload is thought to be advantageous when acquiring pressure-volume loop data because its effects on activating the sympathetic nervous system which impacts on the pressure-volume relationship is minimized.

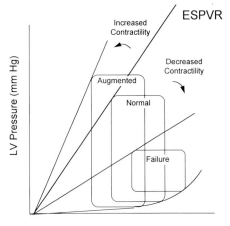

LV Volume (ml)

Figure 9.9. The left ventricular (LV) pressure-volume diagram demonstrating alterations in the end-systolic pressure-volume relationship (ESPVR) to indicate changes in contractility.

Pressure-Area and Pressure-Volume Loop Analysis

The fundamental elements required to perform pressure-volume loop analysis are a pressure signal, a volume signal (or area signal as a substitute), a recording device such as a personal computer or workstation to coordinate and synchronize the timing of the pressure-volume signals, and a loop analysis program with a user interface to edit premature ventricular contractions or other possible signal artifacts. Our group has developed a computer workstation program (Apollo Computer Inc. Model DN3550, Chelmsford, MA) to record and display the pressure-volume loops on-line during data acquisition, and a customized personal computer program (ASYST Software Technologies, Inc., Rochester, NY) to analyze the pressure-volume loops and calculate indices of ventricular performance off-line (Figure 9.10) [28-30]. To accomplish this, the echocardiographic automated border detection system was configured to allow for direct recording of the analog area or volume signal through a customized hardware and software interface, which is now commercially available (Hewlett-Packard, Andover, MA). An analog to digital converter set at 150 Hz was used with an acquisition system (Model RTS-132, Significant, Hudson, MA). An electrocardiographic signal, such as lead II, was used to synchronize the timing of data acquisition. Pressure-volume loops were plotted in real time.

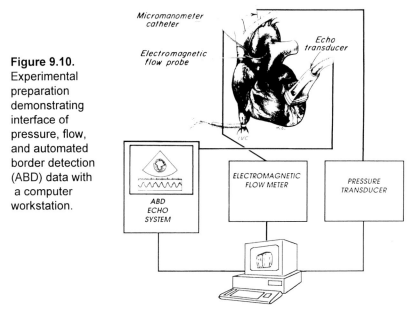

Figure 9.10. Experimental preparation demonstrating interface of pressure, flow, and automated border detection (ABD) data with a computer workstation.

Signal Processing and Timing

All physiologic signals were transferred into a customized personal computer program written in ASYST software off-line. Signals in the loop program were low pass filtered using the inverse Fourier transform of the Blackman window with a cutoff frequency set at 50 Hz to eliminate high frequency noise as previously described [28,29,31]. This filter has been shown not to alter the physiological signal spectrum while suppressing electromagnetic interference. This filtering of echocardiographic automated border detection data may not be necessary with recent refinements in the ultrasound system which have reduced signal noise especially when data are acquired in an environment with little electromagnetic interference. Although the echocardiographic automated border detection system is able to make measurements very quickly, its temporal resolution of approximately 30 Hz may affect the timing of the pressure-volume loop because certain events, such as isovolumic contraction, lasts in less than one 33 msec frame. To correct for this relative delay in echocardiographic area or volume output, the pressure signal was plotted with a variable delay that was adjusted for each loop run by aligning the point immediately preceding isovolumic contraction on the pressure waveform with the first occurrence of maximal area or volume. Further fine adjustments in signal alignment were made by visual inspection of the pressure-volume or pressure-area loop in order to make the isovolumic contraction and relaxation portions of the loop appear vertical. The average amount of delay for 36 inferior vena caval occlusion runs in a canine experiment was 13 ± 19 msec (range 0 to 66 msec).

Calculations of Indices of Ventricular Performance

Established measures of ventricular performance were applied to pressure-volume and pressure-area loops, including end-systolic elastance (E_{es}) or the end-systolic pressure-volume relationship, time-varying elastance (E(t)) for the calculation of maximal elastance (E_{max}), and preload recruitable stroke work (PRSW) or the stroke work - end-diastolic volume relation [22-24]. Pressure-area and pressure-volume loops were analyzed in an identical manner with area simply substituted for volume. Elastance from pressure-area loops was designated E' to differentiate it from the standard symbol E used for pressure-volume analyses. Stroke force was defined as: Pressure d Area, in a manner similar to stroke work, which is: Pressure d Volume. Data sets were divided into cardiac cycles from the R wave of the ECG allowing the user to eliminate ectopic beats. End-systolic elastance was determined as the slope of the maximum pressure/volume points using an automated iterative linear regression method [24,25]. E(t) was derived every 7 msec from linear regression of the isochronous pressure-volume points of differently loaded beats beginning with end-diastole and continuing past end-systole using the equation:

$$E(t) = P(t) / [V(t)-Vo(t)],$$

where E(t) = time-varying elastance, P = pressure, V = volume, t = time, Vo = volume axis intercept. The maximal value of E(t) was defined as maximal elastance or E_{max} [24,25]. E (t) analysis for pressure-area relations was performed using the above identical equation with area substituted for volume (Figure 9.11). Glower *et al.* originally described PRSW or the slope of the stroke work - end-diastolic volume relationship as an index of ventricular contractility which is also predominantly insensitive to loading conditions [25]. Its potential advantage is that it uses information from the entire pressure-volume loop, rather than relying on a series of end-systolic points. Preload recruitable stroke force (PRSF) was calculated in a similar manner from pressure-area loop data as the slope of the stroke force - end-diastolic area relationship.

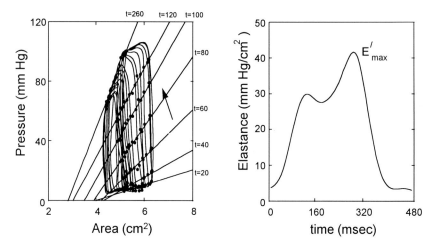

Figure 9.11. An example of the calculation of time-varying elastance from pressure-area loops acquired during inferior vena caval occlusion. The left panel demonstrates sets of isochronous pressure-area points at representative times from the onset of systole. Time (t) is shown in msec. The right panel is the plot of the elastance throughout time with the maximal value shown as E'_{max}. Reprinted with permission from the American College of Cardiology, *J Am Coll Cardiol* 1994;23:242-252.

Validation of Pressure-Area Relations

An animal study was conducted in our laboratory to describe the effects of preload, afterload, and contractility on left ventricular pressure-area relations with on-line cross-sectional area acquired by echocardiographic automated border detection [28]. Eight dogs were instrumented with high fidelity left ventricular pressure catheters and electromagnetic flow probes placed on the ascending aorta. The mid-ventricular short axis plane was used to record echocardiographic automated border detection data. Preload was rapidly altered by inferior vena caval occlusion (Figure 9.12).

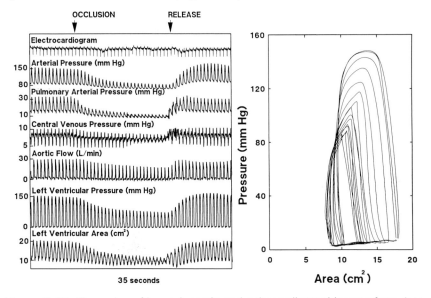

Figure 9.12. Examples of hemodynamic and echocardiographic waveform data and left ventricular pressure-area loops constructed and displayed on-line during inferior vena caval occlusion from a dog model. Waveform data appear on the left, and loop data on the right. Reprinted with permission from the American College of Cardiology, *J Am Coll Cardiol* 1994;23:242-252.

To assess the effects of alterations in afterload on pressure-area relations, pressure-area loops were also recorded during transient descending thoracic aortic occlusion. Pressure-area loops compared favorably with simultaneous pressure-volume loops constructed from LV pressure and LV ejection volume. Similar changes in stroke work $\int PdV$ versus changes in stroke force $\int PdA$ were observed during caval occlusion; r=0.90, SEE=10%. Changes in stroke volume versus changes in stroke area were also correlated for inferior vena caval occlusion and aortic occlusion; r=0.84, SEE=8%. These data demonstrated that pressure-area relations using echocardiographic automated border detection vary in a predominately linear fashion when compared to pressure-volume relations over a wide range of values. Pressure-area relations were then assessed during pharmacological alterations in contractility. Dobutamine was infused as a positive inotropic agent (2-5 µg/kg/min), and propranolol was infused (2-5 mg bolus) as a negative inotropic agent. Left ventricular contractility was assessed by determining $E'es$, E'_{max}, and PRSF as described above. Pressure-area relations demonstrated the physiologically predicted alterations in contractility. Contractility increased with dobutamine (n=7); E'_{es}: 30±11 to 67±24* mmHg/cm² , E'_{max}: 37±11 to 82±26* mmHg/cm² , and PRSF: 81±24 to 197±92* mmHg-cm² (*p<0.02 vs. control). Contractility decreased with propranolol (n = 5); E'_{es}: 20±4 to 13±4** mmHg/cm², E'_{max}: 29±8 to 15±5** mmHg/cm², and PRSF 66±14 to 40±9** (Figures 9.13 and 9.14).

Figure 9.13. Examples of on-line pressure-area loops with end-systolic pressure-area relation-ship shown immediately before (panel A), and with dobutamine infusion (panel B). Panel C: time-varying elastance with maximal elastance (E'_{max}). Panel D: preload recruitable stroke force for the same control and dobutamine loops with a significant increase with dobutamine. Reprinted with permission from the American College of Cardiology, *J Am Coll Cardiol* 1994;23:242-252.

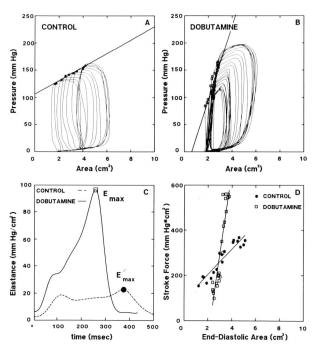

Figure 9.14. Examples of on-line pressure-area loops with end-systolic pressure-area relationship shown immediately before (panel A), and with propranolol infusion (panel B). Panel C: time-varying elastance with maximal elastance (E'_{max}). Panel D: preload recruitable stroke force for the same control and propranolol loops with a significant decrease with propranolol. Reprinted with permission from the American College of Cardiology, *J Am Coll Cardiol* 1994;23:242-252.

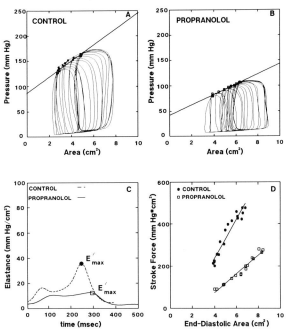

Intraoperative Left Ventricular Pressure-Area Relations

These methods to assess left ventricular performance from pressure-area relations were applied intraoperatively to patients undergoing coronary artery bypass surgery to determine the potential effects of cardiopulmonary bypass on ventricular contractility [29]. Thirteen patients were instrumented with high-fidelity pressure catheters and transesophageal echocardiography to assess pressure-area relations during transient inferior vena caval occlusion. Pressure-area loop studies were performed before and immediately after cardiopulmonary bypass (Figure 9.15).

Complete data sets were available on 7 patients. Estimates of left ventricular performance were made from similar calculations of E'_{es}, E'_{max}, and PRSF described above before and after bypass (Figure 9.16).

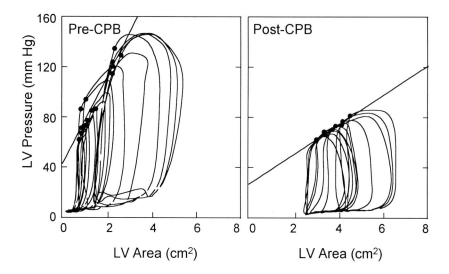

Figure 9.15. An example of pressure-area loops before and immediately after cardiopulmonary bypass (CPB) in a patient undergoing cardiac surgery. Reprinted with permission from the American Heart Association, *Circulation* 1994;89:180-190.

The results of this study performed on a relatively small series of patients demonstrated significant decreases in contractility after bypass as assessed by the load independent indices of ventricular function, where the standard measures of stroke volume, cardiac output, and fractional area change (two-dimensional ejection fraction) were unchanged. This study demonstrates that depression of left ventricular contractility may occur after cardiopulmonary bypass which is thought to be a result of hypothermia and/or ischemia-reperfusion injury [32]. This study also demonstrates that pressure-area relations using transesophageal echocardiography may be applied to the clinical operating room to assess left ventricular contractility.

Arterial Pressure as a Substitute for Left Ventricular Pressure

Although pressure-area relations can be used in the operating room to assess myocardial contractility, these measures have still required the need for instrumentation of the left ventricle with a pressure-sensing catheter. Previous investigators have successfully used central aortic pressure as a substitute for left ventricular ejection pressure [33], and a more recent study was carried out to determine if arterial pressure can be used as a substitute for left ventricular pressure when determining pressure-area relations [34]. We studied thirteen patients before and 8 patients after cardiac surgery with transesophageal echocardiographic automated border detection, high-fidelity left ventricular pressure catheters, and routine fluid-filled femoral arterial pressure catheters. Pressure-area loops were assessed during inferior vena caval occlusions (Figure 9.17).

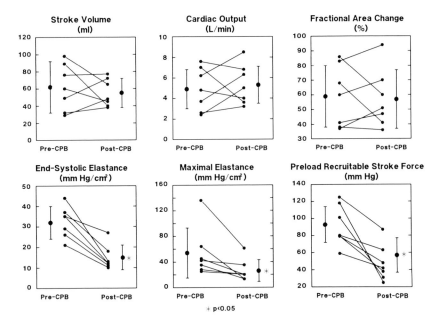

Figure 9.16. Standard and pressure-area indices of left ventricular function from 7 patients before and after cardiopulmonary bypass (CPB). Reprinted with permission from the American Heart Association, *Circulation* 1994;89:180-190.

Technically adequate data were available from 20 studies on 13 patients. A computer program was developed to automatically correct for the delay in the femoral arterial pressure by aligning end-diastolic arterial pressure (minimum pressure) with end-diastolic area (maximal area). Estimates of E'_{es} from LV pressure-area loops correlated with estimates of E'_{es} from femoral arterial pressure *vs* LV area loops (r=0.94, SEE=3 mmHg/cm²). In 7 patients with paired data before and after surgery, similar decreases in E'_{es} using femoral arterial pressure and LV pressure were observed (Figure 9.18). This study extends the application of pressure-volume relations to patients in the operating room without having to additionally instrument the left ventricle with a pressure catheter.

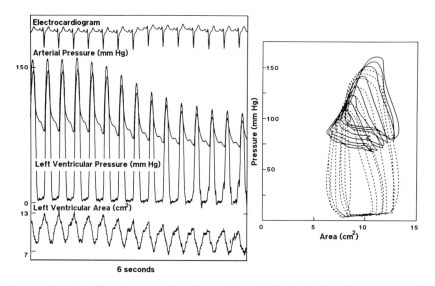

Figure 9.17. Left: An example of waveform data during inferior vena caval occlusion from a patient undergoing coronary bypass surgery. Minimum femoral arterial pressure has been realigned with end-diastolic left ventricular pressure and end-diastolic cross-sectional area. Right: Corresponding simultaneous ventricular pressure-area loops in dashed lines and superimposed arterial pressure-area loops in solid lines. Reprinted with permission from *Anesthesiology* 1994;81:553-562.

Assessment of Right Ventricular Performance

Right ventricular function appears to play an important role in patients with severe heart failure who may be in need of mechanical left ventricular assistance. Assessment of right ventricular contractility has been clinically challenging because its complex geometric shape. Although the concepts of pressure-volume relations have been successfully applied to the right ventricle in the past, there has been no practical means to assess right ventricular volume on-line in a clinical setting [35,36]. The potential for right ventricular cavity area by echocardiographic automated border detection to estimate changes in volume and to assess right ventricular function has been evaluated recently in our laboratory in an isolated canine heart preparation [37]. Eight excised hearts had placement of both right and left intraventricular balloons and were perfused in an ex-vivo apparatus, where biventricular volumes were controlled independently. Right ventricular area data from the level of the left midventricular short-axis plane and pressure data were recorded on a computer workstation. As right ventricular volumes were varied, a predominantly linear relation was observed with right ventricular area: group mean r=0.98 (y=0.16x+0.97, SEE=0.21 cm²) (Figure 9.19).

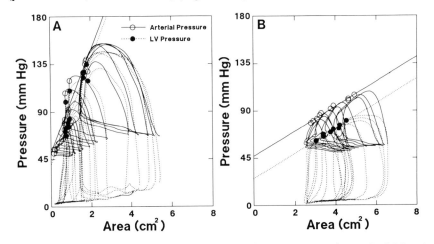

Figure 9.18. Examples of simultaneous arterial pressure-area loops (solid lines) and ventricular pressure-area loops (dashed lines) before (panel A) and immediately after (panel B) cardiopulmonary bypass from the same patient. Left ventricular (LV) pressure E'_{es} decreased from 49 to 12 mmHg/cm², and a similar change occurred with arterial pressure E'_{es} from 50 to 12 mmHg/cm². E'_{es}; end-systolic elastance. Reprinted with permission from *Anesthesiology* 1994;81:553-562.

Alterations in left ventricular volume resulted in a parallel shift of the right ventricular area-volume relationship from interventricular septal shift, although this relationship remained linear. End-systolic pressure-area and pressure-volume relations using simultaneously recorded right ventricular pressure were both highly linear and co-varied with changing left ventricular volume. These data from this animal model support the potential utility of echocardiographic automated border detection to be also used to assess right ventricular function. We have recently acquired preliminary data using transesophageal echocardio-graphic automated border detection and high fidelity pressure to assess intraoperative right ventricular performance in patients undergoing left ventricular assist device implantation (Figure 9.20) [38]. These data on right ventricular contractility demonstrate the potential to utilize this method to aid in the management of these patients with severe congestive heart failure.

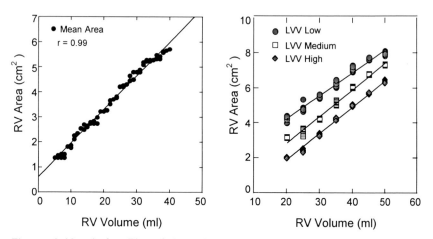

Figure 9.19. Left: Plot of the relationship of right ventricular (RV) cross-sectional area at the mid-ventricular short-axis plane with true RV volume from an isolated canine heart preparation with biventricular balloons. Right: Parallel shift of the RV area-volume relationship with changes in left ventricular volumes (LVV) from septal shifting. Reprinted with permission from the American Heart Association, *Circulation* 1995;92:1026-1033.

Figure 9.20. Right ventricular (RV) pressure-area loops acquired with intraoperative transesophageal automated border detection during inferior vena caval occlusion from a patient with severe congestive heart failure.

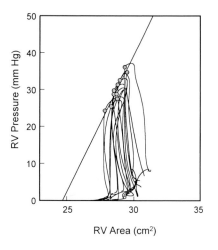

Conclusion

Transesophageal echocardiographic automated border detection has made the application of the important concepts of pressure-volume relations to assess ventricular contractility possible in the operating room. It is appropriate to emphasize that echocardiographic automated border detection in its present form requires high image quality, is highly dependent on operator gain settings, and is sensitive to cardiac translational movements because two-dimensions are used to estimate changes in three-dimensional volume. However, high quality on-line area or volume data may be obtained using intraoperative transesophageal automated border detection and may be combined with either ventricular or femoral arterial pressure to apply concepts of pressure-volume relations as measures of ventricular performance.

References

1. Stewart WJ, Currie PJ, Salcedo EE, Lytle BW, Gill CC, Schiavone WA, Agler DA, Cosgrove DM. Intraoperative Doppler color flow mapping for decision-making in valve repair for mitral regurgitation. Technique and results in 100 patients. *Circulation* 1990;81:556-66.
2. Smith JS, Cahalan MK, Benefiel DJ, Byrd BF, Lurz FW, Shapiro WA, Roizen MF, Bouchard A, Schiller NB. Intraoperative detection of myocardial ischemia in high risk patients: Electrocardiography versus two-dimensional transesophageal echocardiography. *Circulation* 1985;72:1015-1021.
3. Thys DM, Hillel Z, Goldman ME, Mindich BP, Kaplan JA. A comparison for hemodynamic indices by invasive monitoring and two-dimensional echocardiography. *Anesthesiology* 1987;67:630-634.
4. Urbanowitz JH, Shaaban MJ, Cohen NH, Cahalan MK, Botvinick EH, Chatterjee K, Schiller NB, Dae MW, Matthay MA. Comparison of ransesophageal echocardiographic and scintigraphic estimates of left ventricular end-diastolic volume index and ejection fraction in patients following coronary artery bypass grafting. *Anesthesiology* 1990;72:607-612.
5. Perez JE, Waggoner AD, Barzilai B, Melton HE, Miller JG, Sobel BE. On-line assessment of ventricular function by automatic boundary detection and ultrasonic backscatter imaging. *J Am Coll Cardiol* 1992;19:313-320.
6. Vandenberg BF, Rath LS, Stuhlmuller P, Melton HE, Skorton D. Estimation of left ventricular cavity area with an on-line semiautomated echocardiographic edge detection system. *Circulation* 1992;86:159-166.
7. Gorcsan J, Morita S, Mandarino WA, Deneault LG, Kawai A, Kormos RL, Griffith BP, Pinsky MR. Two-dimensional echocardiographic automated border detection

accurately reflects changes in left ventricular volume. *J Am Soc Echocardiogr* 1993;6:482-489.

8. Gorcsan J, Lazar JM, Romand J, Pinsky MR. On-line estimation of stroke volume by means of echocardiographic automated border detection in the canine left ventricle. *Am Heart J* 1993;125:1316-1323.

9. Appleyard RF, Glantz SA. Two-dimensions describe left ventricular volume change during hemodynamic transients. *Am J Physiol* 1990;258:H277-H284.

10. Cahalan MK, Ionescu P, Melton HE, Adler S, Kee LL, Schiller NB. Automated real-time analysis of intraoperative transesophageal echocardiograms: *Anesthesiology* 1993;78:477-485.

11. Gorcsan J, Lazar JM, Schulman DS, Follansbee WP. Comparison of left ventricular function by echocardiographic automated border detection and by radionuclide ejection fraction. *Am J Cardiol* 1993;72:810-815.

12. Cheung AT, Salvino JS, Weiss SJ, Aukburg SJ, Berlin JA. Echocardiographic and hemodynamic indices of left ventricular preload in patients with normal and abnormal ventricular function. *Anesthesiology* 1994;81:376-387.

13. Gorcsan J, Gasior TA, Mandarino WA, Deneault LG, Hattler BG, Pinsky MR. On-line estimation of changes in left ventricular stroke volume by transesophageal echocardiograhic automated border detection in patients undergoing coronary artery bypass grafting. *Am J Cardiol* 1993;72:721-727.

14. Schiller NB, Shah PM, Crawford M, Demaria A, Devereaux R, Feigenbaum H, Gutgesell H, Reichek N, Sahn D, Schnittger I. Recommendations for quantitation of the left ventricle by two-dimensional echocardiography. *J Am Soc Echocardiogr* 1989;2:358-367.

15. Smith MD, MacPhail B, Harrison MR, Lenhoff SJ, DeMaria AN. Value and limitations of transesophageal echocardiography in determination of left ventricular volumes and ejection fraction. *J Am Coll Cardiol* 1992;19:1213-1222.

16. Hozumi T, Shakudo M, Shah PM. Quantitation of left ventricular volumes and ejection fraction biplane transesophageal echocardiography. *Am J Cardiol* 1993;72:356-359.

17. Morrissey RL, Siu SC, Guerrero JL, Newell JB, Weyman AE, Picard MH. Automated assessment of ventricular volume and function by echocardiography: Validation of automated border detection. *J Am Soc Echocardiogr* 1994;7:107-115.

18. Katz W, Gasior TA, Reddy SBC, Gorcsan J. Utility and limitations of biplane transesophageal echocardiographic automated border detection for estimation of left ventricular stroke volume and cardiac output. *Am Heart J* 1994;128:389-396.

19. Gorcsan J, Denault A, Mandarino WA, Pinsky MR. Left ventricular pressure-volume relations with transesophageal echocardiographic automated border detection: Comparison with conductance catheter technique. *Am Heart J* 1996;131:544-552.

20. Baan J, Van Der Velde ET, DeBruin HG, Smeenk GJ, Koops, Van Dijk AD, Temmerman D, Senden J, Bruis B. Continuous measurement of left ventricular volume in animals and humans by conductance catheter. *Circulation* 1984;5:812-823.

21. Kass DA, Yamazaki T, Burkhoff D, Maughan WL, Sagawa K. Determination of left ventricular end-systolic pressure-volume relationships by the conductance (volume) catheter technique. *Circulation* 1986;3:586-595.
22. Bland JM, Altman DG. Statistical methods for assessing agreement between two methods of clinical measurement. *Lancet* 1986;1:307-310.
23. Suga H, Sagawa K, Shoukas. Load independence of the instantaneous pressure-volume ratio of the canine left ventricle and effects of epinephrine and heart rate on the ratio. *Circ Res* 1973;32:314-322.
24. Suga H, Sagawa K. Instantaneous pressure-volume relationships and their ratio in the excised, supported canine left ventricle. *Circ Res* 1974;35:117-126.
25. Glower DD, Spratt, JA, Snow ND, Kabas JS, Davis JW, Olsen CO, Tyson GS, Sabiston DC, Rankin JS. Linearity of the Frank-Starling relationship in the intact heart: the concept of preload recruitable stroke work. *Circulation* 1985;5:994-1009.
26. Baan J, Van Der Velde ET. Sensitivity of left ventricular end-systolic pressure-volume elation to type of loading intervention in dogs. *Circ Res* 1988;62:1247-1258.
27. Kass DA, Yamazaki T, Burkhoff D, Maughan WL, Sagawa K. Determination of left ventricular end-systolic pressure-volume relationships by the conductance (volume) catheter technique. *Circulation* 1986;73:586-595.
28. Gorcsan J, Romand JA, Mandarino WA, Deneault LG, Pinsky MR. Assessment of left ventricular performance by on-line pressure-area relations using echocardiographic automated border detection. *J Am Coll Cardiol* 1994;23:242-252.
29. Gorcsan J, Gasior TA, Mandarino WA, Deneault LG, Hattler BG, Pinsky MR. Assessment of the immediate effects of cardiopulmonary bypass on left ventricular performance by on-line pressure-area relations. *Circulation* 1994;89:180-190.
30. Deneault LG, Kancel MJ, Denault A, Mandarino WA, Gasior TA, Gorcsan J, Pinsky MR. A system for the on-line acquisition, visualization, and analysis of pressure-area loops. *Comp Biomed Res* 1994;27:61-67.
31. Blackman RB, Tukey JW: *The Measurement of Power Spectra*. New York, NY: Dover Publications, 1958;129-135.
32. Breissblatt WM, Stein KL, Wolfe CJ. Acute myocardial dysfunction and recovery: A common occurrence after coronary bypass surgery. *J Am Coll Cardiol* 1990;15:1261-1269.
33. Grossman W, Braunwald E, Mann T, McLaurin LP, Green LH. Contractile state of the left ventricle in man as evaluated from end-systolic pressure-volume relations. *Circulation* 1977;56:845-852.
34. Gorcsan J, Denault A, Gasior TA, Mandarino WH, Kancel MJ, Deneault LG, Hattler BG, Pinsky MR. Rapid estimation of left ventricular contractility from end-systolic relations by echocardiographic automated border detection and femoral arterial pressure. *Anesthesiology* 1994;81:553-562
35. Maughan WL, Shoukas AA, Sagawa K, Weisfeldt ML. Instantaneous pressure-volume relationship of the canine right ventricle. *Circ Res* 1979;44:309-315.
36. Karunanithi MK, Michniewicz J, Copeland SE, Feneley MP. Right ventricular preload recruitable stroke work, end-systolic pressure-volume, and dp/dtmax-end-

diastolic volume relations compared as indexes of right ventricular contractile performance in conscious dogs. *Circ Res* 1992;70:1169-1179.

37. Oe M, Gorcsan J, Mandarino WA, Kawai A, Griffith BP, Kormos RL. Automated echocardiographic measures of right ventricular area as an index of volume and end-systolic pressure-area relations to assess right ventricular function. *Circulation* 1995;92:1026-1033.

38. Kormos RL, Mandarino WA, Gasior TA, Griffith BP, Gorcsan J. Assessment of the immediate effects of mechanical left ventricular assistance on right ventricular performance by automated pressure-area relations. *J Am Coll Cardiol* 1995;25:150A (Abstract).

10 Color Kinesis: One Step Beyond Acoustic Quantification

Victor Mor-Avi and Roberto M. Lang

Two-dimensional echocardiography is currently the most widely used noninvasive imaging modality for the evaluation of left ventricular function due to its ability to depict myocardial wall motion in real time. Conventional clinical assessment of regional wall motion abnormalities is based on visual interpretation of the magnitude of systolic endocardial excursion and wall thickening. However, this method is highly subjective and skill-dependent, particularly during the interpretation of stress echocardiographic studies. Consequently, variety of quantitative techniques for objective analysis of left ventricular endocardial motion have been developed [1-10]. Prior to the development of acoustic quantification [11-15], these techniques were mostly based on manual off-line frame-by-frame tracing of the myocardial boundaries. Since it is often difficult to accurately define the endocardial and epicardial borders, these time-consuming methods remain subjective and impractical for routine clinical use., Accordingly, a variety of computerized methods of edge detection have been recently developed [8,16-20]. Although automated to a greater extent, these methods still require off-line processing. The development of acoustic quantification provided a partial solution to these difficulties, since it allowed automated detection of the endocardial border, thereby eliminating the need for manual tracing of multiple frames. This method allows real time acquisition of continuous signals reflecting left ventricular cross-sectional area or volume throughout the cardiac cycle [12,13,21]. However, these signals reflect global rather than regional left ventricular performance. The ability to easily assess regional systolic and diastolic function could provide useful information in a variety of clinical states, including coronary artery disease.

To facilitate a more objective evaluation of regional left ventricular performance, Color Kinesis, a new real-time technique based on acoustic quantification, has been developed and incorporated into a commercial ultrasound system (see Chapter 1). This technique compares tissue backscatter values between successive acoustic frames, and detects pixel transitions between blood and myocardial tissue throughout systole or diastole. Different color hues are used to color-encode these pixel transitions over time, and overlaid on the two-dimensional images. Colors are added one per frame and accumulate throughout systole or diastole. Thus, a single end-systolic or end-diastolic frame provides an integrated display reflecting the magnitude and timing of endocardial motion throughout the ejection or filling period of the most recent cardiac cycle. This chapter will initially describe in more detail the basic features of Color Kinesis and its principles of operation.

The validation of new technologies is of primary importance prior to routine clinical use. However, Color Kinesis is based on exactly the same principles used by acoustic quantification to differentiate myocardial tissue from blood. Color Kinesis basically differs from acoustic quantification only in the way this information is used to track and display endocardial motion. In this regard, Color Kinesis data may be considered as an extension of acoustic quantification, which has been previously extensively validated against different techniques by numerous investigators [13-15,21-26].

The feasibility of accurately tracking the endocardial motion with Color Kinesis in normal subjects and in patients with regional wall motion abnormalities has been recently established by several investigators [27-29]. However, similar to acoustic quantification, the identification of the endocardial boundary with Color Kinesis is a threshold technique based on operator dependent gain settings. As a result, acquisition of Color Kinesis images requires understanding of the principles of operation of this technology, as well as awareness of the pitfalls and potential difficulties. Accordingly, guidelines for the acquisition of technically adequate color-encoding of the endocardial motion will also be briefly described below.

Theoretically, with appropriate methods of analysis, end-systolic and end-diastolic Color Kinesis images could provide easy and objective evaluation of endocardial motion, both on a global and regional basis. Accordingly, we will describe in detail the recently developed method of quantitative segmental analysis of Color Kinesis images. This technique is based on counting colored pixels and using the pixel counts to calculate indices reflecting the magnitude and timing of systolic and diastolic left ventricular endocardial motion.

In this chapter, we will also describe the patterns of regional systolic and diastolic endocardial excursion obtained using our automated technique of analysis in a group of normal subjects. We will then describe how these normal patterns can be used as a reference for comparison to objectively detect regional wall motion abnormalities [29], in the following chapter where the potential clinical applications of these analysis techniques will be surveyed.

Abnormal temporal characteristics of regional endocardial motion during systole and diastole have been previously shown to reflect myocardial ischemia [30-34]. These phase abnormalities were evident before reduced magnitude of motion was noted. However, visual assessment of the temporal characteristics of endocardial motion is virtually impossible even for experienced readers. Due to the lack of easy techniques of analysis, the timing of endocardial motion has been so far disregarded in the clinical practice. Color Kinesis provides for an opportunity for easy and objective assessment of the temporal characteristics of the endocardial motion on a regional basis, which can be quantified by decoding the end-systolic and end-diastolic color overlays.

We will briefly summarize our results regarding the quantification of the temporal sequences of contraction and relaxation in normal subjects, and describe how the temporal indices of regional myocardial function are affected by different pharmacological agents. The next chapter will present clinical data demonstrating the differences in temporal sequences of contraction between (1) normal myocardial segments, (2) ischemic segments with preserved magnitude of motion, and (3) segments with reduced motion.

Principles of Operation

Color Kinesis processes the ultrasound backscatter data and generates for each acoustic frame a binary blood/tissue mask image, where each pixel is classified as either blood or myocardial tissue. The system detects pixel value transitions between blood and tissue in this mask image on a frame-by-frame basis, and uses color-encoding to mark these transitions over time. The color information is displayed in real time as an overlay superimposed on the two-dimensional echocardiographic image. The color overlay is continuously updated by adding one specific color hue per frame (Figure 10.1). Colors accumulate throughout systole or diastole, depending on which mode of operation is selected, and are removed before the beginning of the next cardiac cycle. Thus, the end-systolic or end-diastolic color overlay provides an integrated display of the magnitude and timing of endocardial excursion of the most recent heart beat (Figure 10.2).

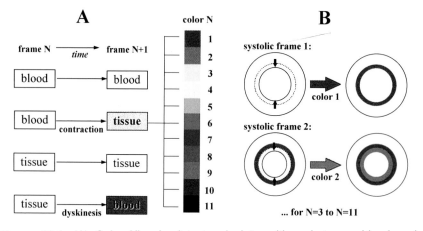

Figure 10.1. (A) Color Kinesis detects pixel transitions between blood and myocardial tissue on a frame by frame basis. In systole, pixels that change from blood to tissue are color-encoded using up to 11 distinct colors (color bar in the middle). Optional encoding with a specific color hue different from all colors used to encode normal endocardial motion can be be applied to pixels that show paradoxical transition from tissue to blood. (B) Schematic representation of the frame by frame color-encoding during systolic contraction in the short axis view.

Color Kinesis locks the imaging frame rate at 30 Hz. Thus, each frame represents a constant time interval of 33 ms. The timing of color-encoding is determined as follows. Color encoding of systolic contraction is triggered by the R-wave of the electrocardiogram. The duration of the systolic ejection time (ET, in ms) is calculated using the following empirical formula:

$$ET = \frac{346}{\sqrt{HR}}$$

(1)

where HR is heart rate in beats per second. Color-encoding of diastole starts at end-systole and ends either a fixed number of frames later (corresponding to the maximal number of colors available, which is currently 19), or at the ensuing R-wave, whichever occurs first.

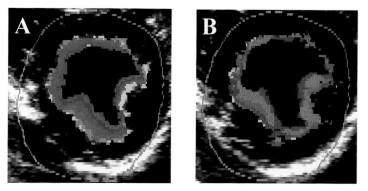

Figure 10.2. Example of normal end-systolic (left) and end-diastolic (right) images obtained with Color Kinesis in the parasternal short axis view.

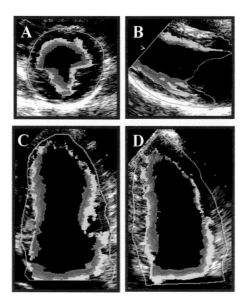

Figure 10.3. End-systolic Color Kinesis images obtained in a normal subject in four standard echocardiographic views: (A) parasternal short axis, (B) parasternal long axis, (C) apical four-chamber, and (D) apical two-chamber view.

Color Kinesis imaging can be obtained in any view using either the transthoracic (Figure 10.3) or transesophageal approach. Ideally, Color Kinesis image sequences should be stored digitally on optical disk to avoid image degradation which occurs while using videotapes.

An additional feature of Color Kinesis is its ability to color-encode paradoxical pixel transitions, *i.e.* transitions from tissue to blood during systole or from blood to tissue during diastole. These pixel transitions are color-encoded using a specific hue, which is different from colors used to encode normal endocardial motion (Figure 10.4). This feature is called 'dyskinesis' and its display is optional (see Chapter 1). However, the classification of paradoxical pixel transitions is performed by the system regardless of whether the 'dyskinesis' mode is activated, and the 'dyskinetic' display can be toggled on or off during playback of digitally stored image sequences.

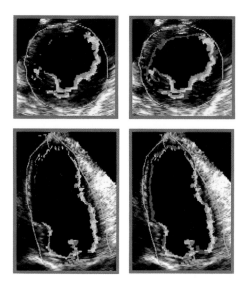

Figure 10.4. Example of short axis (top) and apical four-chamber (bottom) Color Kinesis images obtained in a patient with septal regional wall motion abnormality: the lack of colors in the septal segments (left panels) depicts akinetic septum. With the display of paradoxical pixel transitions from tissue to blood activated (right panels, red color), the dyskinetic motion of the septum becomes evident.

Acquisition Techniques

Optimization of Endocardial Tracking

Color Kinesis relies on adequate endocardial definition in order to accurately track the blood-tissue interface. Accordingly, obtaining a two-dimensional image optimized for endocardial definition is a crucial step in performing a technically adequate study. Prior to acquisition of Color Kinesis images, it is recommended to carefully optimize tracking of the endocardial boundary with acoustic quantification [35]. Once Color Kinesis is activated, endocardial tracking should be reconfirmed by toggling the color-encoding on and off. Color Kinesis tracking can be graded as good, usable, or technically inadequate. Good tracking demonstrates consistent, smooth, continuous, and concentric layers of color that accurately track endocardial boundaries. Usable tracking differs from good in that scattered spots of colors are noted within the image, but Color Kinesis still reflects endocardial motion for most of the left ventricle. Technically inadequate tracking results in "bleeding" of colors with a significant number of color spots due to poor image quality. In these cases, endocardial motion is not accurately represented. At times, fine adjustments of the time-gain compensation settings and lateral gain controls may be required to optimize regional Color Kinesis tracking. However, if changes are made in the Color Kinesis mode, the operator should return to the acoustic quantification mode to verify adequate tracking of the endocardial boundaries.

Ensuring Proper Timing of Acquisition

It is crucial to ensure that the timing of color encoding accurately corresponds to that of left ventricular contraction or relaxation. In the absence of pharmacologic interventions, the empirical formula used to calculate the duration of the systolic ejection time (equation 1) is generally accurate. However, inaccurate identification of the onset of diastole may result in misleading data, because endocardial expansion that occurs during the initial rapid filling phase of diastole is not color-encoded. Therefore, verification of the accuracy of the default settings is of particular importance when acquiring diastolic Color Kinesis images. This can be performed by visually inspecting a Color Kinesis sequence frame-by-frame and by toggling the CK overlay on and off, and is easier to perform in an apical imaging plane since the opening and closing of the mitral valve provide additional timing cues. During systolic Color Kinesis, the first frame to be color-encoded should contain the first two-dimensional image that demonstrates concentric contraction as compared to the previous frame. Similarly, the first diastolic frame to be color-encoded should contain the first two-dimensional image demonstrating concentric expansion after the smallest left ventricular area is observed. The last color-encoded diastolic frame should correspond to the largest left ventricular area. If a timing problem is noted, the start and duration times should be adjusted to ensure that color-encoding begins and ends at the appropriate times.

Methods of Analysis

In this section we will describe the methods of analysis we have applied to Color Kinesis images obtained in the parasternal short axis and apical four-chamber views. These methods were implemented in a custom designed image processing software written for a personal computer. Initially, two important issues had to be addressed. First, should a floating frame of reference be used to compensate for possible cardiac translation or rotation? And second, which segmentation schemes would best match endocardial motion throughout the cardiac cycle, while correctly reflecting the coronary perfusion territories?

Choice of Frame of Reference

Whereas some investigators have demonstrated advantages of a floating over fixed reference frame [2,36,37], others have not found significant differences between these methods [4,38]. Different methodologies of image alignment using a floating reference have been utilized to correct for cardiac translation and rotation that may occur during the cardiac cycle. These methods have predominantly used the centroid of either the endocardial boundary or the entire left ventricular cavity [1,4,19], or other points [2,39] as stationary points for image alignment.

We chose a fixed reference system to analyze end-systolic and end-diastolic Color Kinesis images. This choise was made because Color Kinesis compares identical pixels in successive acoustic frames to identify pixel transitions. In other words, a fixed frame of reference is used at the time that Color Kinesis images are created. Moreover, since each pixel in the color overlay cannot be assigned more than one value, information regarding multiple pixel transitions resulting from translation and rotation is not reflected in the end-systolic or end-diastolic color overlays. Consequently, although a floating reference frame analysis could be applied off-line to end-systolic and end-diastolic Color Kinesis images, this analysis would not necessarily provide a correction for translation and rotation artifacts.

Segmentation Models and Pixel Statistics

Schemes used to segment the left ventricle in the different views should address two issues. First, since regional wall motion abnormalities usually reflect epicardial coronary artery stenosis, segmentation models should reflect the different anatomic perfusion territories. Accordingly, we followed the segmentation schemes described in the guidelines of the American Society of Echocardiography [40]. Implementation of these schemes in our automated digital image analysis required detailed decisions regarding the origin of segmentation, as well as size and geometry of each individual segment.

Segmentation of both short axis and apical four-chamber views originated from the end-systolic left ventricular cavity area centroid, which was previously shown to provide more reproducible data as compared to the centroid of the left ventricular boundary [37]. Cavity centroid was defined by its $x_{1,2}$ coordinates as follows:

$$x_{1,2}(centroid) = \frac{\iint\limits_{S} x \, dx_1 dx_2}{\iint\limits_{S} dx_1 dx_2} \qquad (2)$$

where S is the end-systolic left ventricular cavity area. The zero line was defined by the centroid and a manually determined anatomic landmark represented by the junction between the right ventricular posterior wall endocardium and the inter-ventricular septum [3,5,19,41,42] (Figure 10.5,A). This anatomic landmark was chosen because it was previously shown to be minimally affected by cardiac rotation and translation at rest [42]. The left ventricle was divided into six 60° wedge-shaped sectors.

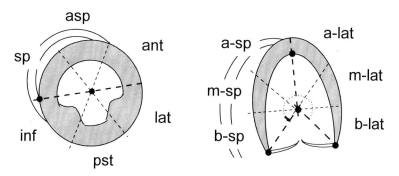

Figure 10.5. Segmentation schemes used for the quantitative segmental analysis of endocardial wall motion (see text for details). Short axis view (SAX, left): ant = anterior, asp = anteroseptal, sp = septal, inf = inferior, pst = posterior, lat = lateral. Apical four-chamber view (A4C, right): b-lat = basal lateral, m-lat = mid-lateral, a-lat = apical-lateral, a-sp = apical-septal, m-sp = mid-septal, b-sp = basal-septal.

In the apical four-chamber view, each image was initially divided into two sections separated by a line (defined as the long axis) connecting the manually determined distal apical endocardium with the calculated end-systolic left ventricular cavity centroid (equation 2). In each section, a wedge-shaped sector was defined between the aforementioned long axis and a line connecting the centroid with the manually determined base of both mitral valve leaflets. This scheme excluded mitral valve motion from the analysis and minimized the variability introduced by individual differences in left ventricular orientation. Each sector was then divided into 3 equiangled sectors. This procedure resulted in a total of 6 sectors originating from the cavity centroid (Figure 10.5,B).

Another important issue related to the design of segmentation models is that the geometry of individual segments should match the regional patterns of endocardial motion. To allow reliable analysis of endocardial motion on a regional basis, each segment must reflect the motion of the corresponding anatomic endocardial segment. To this effect, segmentation lines should ideally be parallel to regional velocity vectors in each frame. Thus, in the short axis view, a radial segmentation scheme provided a simple solution to follow the fairly symmetric radial motion that occurs during normal left ventricular contraction and relaxation. In the apical four-chamber view, endocardial motion has been previously described as inward motion (related to wall thickening), with simultaneous basal motion towards the apex (secondary to long axis shortening) [43,44], which has been described as gradually decreasing from base to apex. To follow this complex motion pattern, segmentation lines should be drawn almost perpendicular to the long axis with a slight angulation towards the apex, which should decrease from base to apex. Implementation of such a non-concentric segmentation model would be considerably more difficult than a simple concentric segmentation. Accordingly, a segmentation scheme originating from a single well-defined point, the left ventricular cavity centroid, was adopted. In fact, the simple concentric and complex non-concentric schemes would result in similar individual segment geometry, with the exception of the boundaries between the apical and mid-ventricular segments.

Following segmentation, pixels of each color and pixels marked as blood were counted in each segment. These pixel counts were subsequently used for the objective assessment of the magnitude and timing of regional endocardial motion during systole and diastole. The magnitude of regional endocardial motion was expressed in terms of the following characteristics: incremental fractional area change (in percent of segmental and global end-diastolic area), endocardial wall displacement (in mm), and fractional radial shortening (in percent of end-diastolic radial dimension). The temporal characteristics of regional endocardial motion were assessed using: incremental and integrated fractional area change and integrated fractional radial shortening as a function of time, as well as mean time of ejection and filling. Analysis techniques used to calculate each of these parameters are described in detail below.

Analysis of Magnitude of Endocardial Motion

Incremental Fractional Area Change

In each segment, for both end-systolic and end-diastolic frames, the number of pixels of each color represents the incremental area change that occurred during the time frame corresponding to that specific color (33 msec period). The end-diastolic area of each individual segment is represented by the total pixel count, *i.e.* all colored pixels and those marked as blood. Normalization of the incremental area change by the end-diastolic area of the corresponding segment results in regional fractional area change (in percent of end-diastolic area of that specific segment). Incremental area changes in all segments were displayed as a stacked color histogram, wherein each time frame is represented by a specific color identical to that used in the Color Kinesis images.

A histogram was also generated for fractional area change in percent of global, end-diastolic area. For this purpose, global end-diastolic area was calculated as the sum of segmental end-diastolic areas in all six segments obtained as described above. The total area of this histogram reflects global fractional area change.

Incremental Endocardial Displacement

To evaluate regional endocardial radial displacement for each time frame, arc approximation was used. The displacement, Δr, was calculated as the radial dimension of a respective color band, according to the following expression:

$$\Delta r = r_{long} - r_{short} = \sqrt{\frac{2A_{long}}{\theta}} - \sqrt{\frac{2A_{short}}{\theta}} \tag{3}$$

where r_{long} and r_{short} are the radial distances from the centroid, A_{long} and A_{short} are the corresponding sector areas, and θ is the sector angle (in radians). This formula was derived from the expression for an area of a sector with radius r:

$$A = \frac{\theta}{2\pi} \cdot \pi r^2 \qquad (4)$$

To obtain the displacement in metric units, areas A_{long} and A_{short} needed to be expressed in cm² rather than pixel counts. Thus, each area was computed as a product of the corresponding pixel count with single pixel area, based on the 5:4 horizontal to vertical aspect ratio (NTSC standard) and imaging depth D (in cm) per 350 pixels:

$$A = pixels \cdot \frac{5}{4} \left(\frac{D}{350} \right)^2 \frac{cm^2}{pixel} \qquad (5)$$

This conversion from pixels to metric units was performed for each consecutive color band in each segment, resulting in approximate endocardial wall displacement during each consecutive time frame. This parameter was also displayed as a stacked color histogram wherein each color represents a specific time during systole or diastole.

Incremental Fractional Radial Shortening

In each segment, fractional radial shortening was also calculated for each time frame, using equation (3), based on the area of the corresponding color band. To evaluate shortening in percent of end-diastolic radial dimension, wall displacement was normalized by segmental end-diastolic radius and multiplied by 100. The results were displayed as a color-encoded stacked histogram.

Phase Analysis of Endocardial Motion

Ejection and Filling Rate

To directly assess the temporal patterns of left ventricular contraction and relaxation, parameters of endocardial motion were displayed as a function of time. Fractional area change was normalized by the 33 msec sampling interval. This normalization resulted in ejection or filling rate (in end-diastolic area per second), which was plotted versus time with data from different segments displayed as stacked time-histograms. This display allowed immediate identification of the magnitude and timing of peak ejection and filling.

Mean Time of Ejection and Filling

For each segment, mean time required for a pixel to change its tissue/blood attribute, which represents the mean time of left ventricular ejection and filling, was calculated from this data as follows:

$$\bar{t} = \frac{\int\limits_{t=0}^{T} t \cdot RFAC(t)dt}{\int\limits_{t=0}^{T} RFAC(t)dt} \tag{6}$$

where $RFAC(t)$ is a function of time representing regional fractional area change, time $t=0$ represents beginning of ejection or filling, and T is total ejection or filling time.

Integrated Fractional Area Change

Time curves reflecting fractional area change for the entire left ventricle integrated with respect to time were constructed to allow quantification of global left ventricular function. This curve provided a simple display of the temporal progression of ejection and filling phases, as well as the total fractional area change at the completion of contraction or relaxation, respectively.

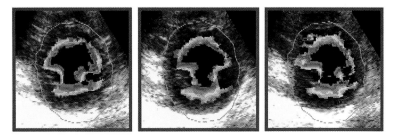

Figure 10.6. Eaxmple of three non-consecutive short axis images obtained in one normal subject for the analysis of reproducibility.

Normalized Regional Time Curves

To facilitate the evaluation of the temporal patterns of contraction and relaxation on a segmental basis, regional time curves reflecting area change and radial shortening, integrated with respect to time and normalized to 100%, were constructed for each segment. To allow intra- and inter-subject comparisons, the effects of heart rate on the duration of contraction and relaxation were eliminated by using linear interpolation to obtain 20 values of each parameter in 5% increments of contraction or relaxation time. Using this display, each curve reaches 100% ejection or filling at 100% systolic or diastolic time, respectively.

Reproducibility

Reproducibility (intra-subject variability) of the segmental analysis of Color Kinesis images was evaluated in a group of 9 randomly selected normal subjects by acquiring and analyzing 3 non-consecutive end-systolic color-encoded images. Reproducibility was quantified for each subject by averaging the regional fractional area change histograms of these 3 repeated measurements and calculating for each segment the standard deviation divided by the mean. Using this strategy of repeated data acquisition and analysis (Figure 10.6), we found the patterns of regional endocardial excursion obtained with Color Kinesis highly consistent. Repeated analyses of non-consecutive Color Kinesis images were found to be reproducible within 11±4% in the short axis view and 12±2% in the apical four-chamber view. Detailed summary of intra-subject variability data for each segment (mean and range) is shown in Figure 10.7. Thus, the reproducibility of this technique proved to be similar to that of other techniques based on manual tracing of endocardial border [4,5].

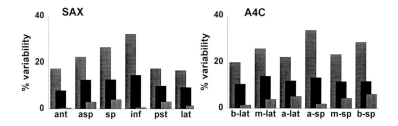

Figure 10.7. Reproducibility of segmental analysis of Color Kinesis images was tested by repeated data acquisitions and analyses. Percent of variability was calculated for each segment as the standard deviation of the repeated measurements divided by their mean. Data is presented as mean of normal subjects (solid bars) together with the extreme values (dashed bars). Modified with permission from the American Heart Association, *Circulation* 1996; 93:1877–1888.

Normal Patterns of LV Contraction and Relaxation

Figures 10.8 to 10.14 show the results of our initial measurements of regional left ventricular systolic and diastolic performance obtained in a group of 12 normal subjects (mean age: 34±5 years) selected based on the high quality of their echocardiographic images.

Normal Magnitude of Endocardial Motion

Figure 10.8 shows stacked color histograms reflecting the incremental area change in each segment during systole (left) and diastole (right). Color hues correspond to those used in Color Kinesis images. In each view, the patterns of endocardial motion during contraction (left) and relaxation (right) were found to be similar. These patterns were more symmetric in the short axis view compared to the apical four-chamber view. In this latter view, reduced endocardial motion was demonstrated in the apical-lateral segment, probably due to poor visualization and tracking of the endocardial border in this region.

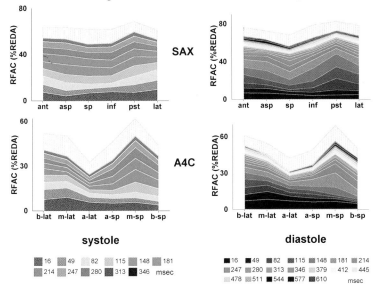

Figure 10.8. Regional incremental fractional area change (RFAC) during systole (left) and diastole (right) in percent of regional end-diastolic area (REDA) in the short axis (SAX, top) and apical four-chamber (A4C, bottom) views. Color encoding schemes are shown at the bottom. Data represent the average of 12 normal subjects; standard deviations are shown as a dashed band.

Incremental area change in percent of global (rather than segmental) left ventricular end-diastolic area also showed similar patterns of motion during contraction (Figure 10.9, left) and relaxation (right) in each view, but with more inter-segmental variability. This increased variability reflects the fact that normalization by a global parameter identical for all segments (such as end-diastolic area of the entire left ventricular cavity), fails to eliminate inter-segmental differences in the geometry and the distances from the centroid. These differences, coupled with true regional variations in the magnitude of endocardial motion, probably account for the peaks observed in the posterior segment (short axis view, Figure 10.9, top), and, basal and apical segments (apical four-chamber view, Figure 10.9, bottom). Thus, it appears that normalization by a regional parameter (such as segmental end diastolic area) is advantageous, because it allows inter-segmental comparisons and eliminates inter-segmental geometrical differences.

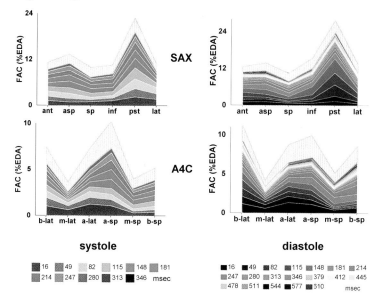

Figure 10.9. Incremental fractional area change (FAC) during systole (left) and diastole (right) in percent of global (rather than regional) left ventricular end-diastolic area (EDA) in the short axis (SAX, top) and apical four-chamber (A4C, bottom) views. Color encoding schemes are shown at the bottom, region notations as in figure 10.5. Data represent the average of 12 normal subjects; standard deviations are shown as a dashed band.

Endocardial wall displacement (Figure 10.10) resulted in patterns of contraction and relaxation similar to those depicted in Figure 10.9, but with less inter-segmental variability. Another difference between these two data sets was the increased contribution of late colors during systole and early colors during diastole to overall wall displacement (Figure 10.10). This is probably because absolute endocardial displacement in mm is less affected by variations in radial distance from the centroid during contraction or relaxation. Although this parameter supposedly provides an absolute measurement of wall motion, and therefore should not be affected by the specific segmental geometry. It should be pointed out that in this study, endocardial displacement was calculated using an arc approximation for each color band. The validity of this approach varies from segment to segment. In particular, this geometric assumption may fail in the short axis view in the inferior, posterior and lateral segments which contain the papillary muscles, as well as in the mid-ventricular and basal segments in the apical four-chamber view. It therefore seems that more specific modeling of the regional endocardial boundary geometry is required before reliable measurements of endocardial wall displacement can be obtained.

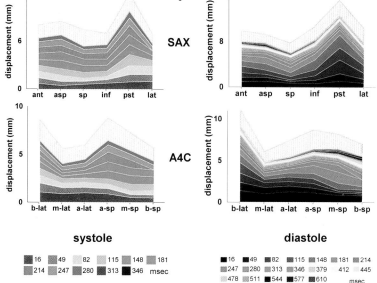

Figure 10.10. Regional endocardial wall displacement during systole (left) and diastole (right) in mm in the short axis (SAX, top) and apical four-chamber (A4C, bottom) views. Color encoding schemes are shown at the bottom, region notations as in figure 5. Data represent the average of 12 normal subjects; standard deviations are shown as a dashed band.

The patterns of fractional radial shortening were almost identical to those reflecting segmental fractional area change (Figure 10.8), because these two parameters are closely related and computed using regional normalization. It is therefore not surprising that fractional radial shortening has a more uniform normal patterns of contraction and relaxation compared to wall displacement.

The patterns of regional endocardial excursion obtained with Color Kinesis were highly consistent in normal subjects. The inter-subject variability of the segmental analysis reflected individual differences in left ventricular chamber geometry and function. The inter-subject variability of each parameter expressed as standard deviation divided by the mean of all subjects, indicates that the short axis view provides more consistent measurements during both contraction and relaxation, when compared to the apical four-chamber view (Table 10.1, columns 1 and 2 versus columns 3 and 4). In both views, fractional area change in percent of segmental end-diastolic area, was found not only to best reflect the uniform pattern of regional endocardial motion, but also provide the most consistent inter-subject measurements (Table 10.1). Based on the results of this study and within the limitations of the specific methods of analysis used, this latter index appears to provide the most reliable picture of the magnitude of regional endocardial wall motion.

Table 10.1. Inter-subject variability: standard deviation in percent of the mean, averaged for all segments in each imaging plane. Abbreviations: RFAC - regional fractional area change, FAC - fractional area change, displ. - displacement, RFS - regional fractional radial shortening.

	SAX		A4C	
	systole	diastole	systole	diastole
RFAC	19	17	29	25
FAC	23	25	37	33
displ.	27	28	35	30
RFS	23	22	33	29

Normal Temporal Sequence of Endocardial Motion

Figures 10.11 to 10.14 present the results of the quantification of the temporal sequences of left ventricular contraction and relaxation. Plots of ejection and filling rates versus time showed major differences between contraction and relaxation, while being similar between views in both systole and diastole (Figure 10.11). The morphology of the plots closely resembled that of time-derivatives of signal-averaged acoustic quantification left ventricular area waveforms [45], as well as data obtained with radionuclide ventriculography [46]. The mean time of contraction was 135±11 msec in the short axis and 133±9 in the apical four-chamber view. The time to peak filling rate was 143±38 and 181±27 msec, in the short axis and the apical four-chamber views, respectively. The mean time of filling was 198±26 msec in the short axis and 195±19 in the apical view.

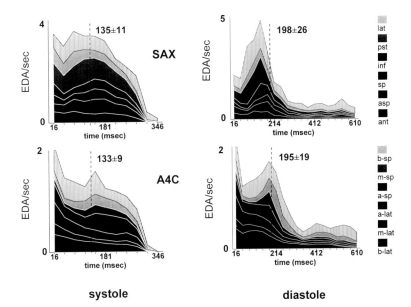

Figure 10.11. Plots of left ventricular ejection rate (left) and filling rate (right) as a function of time in units of global end-diastolic left ventricular area (EDA) per second in the short axis (top) and apical four-chamber (bottom) views. Data from different segments is displayed as stacked time-histograms, and represents the average of 12 normal subjects; mean time of ejection or filling is shown on each plot as a dashed vertical line.

Regional mean time of ejection and filling was found to be uniform in the short axis view (Figure 10.12, top). In contrast, more pronounced inter-segmental variability was observed in the apical four-chamber view (Figure 10.12, bottom). The mean time of both ejection and filling appeared to be longer for septal compared to lateral segments. This parameter, if normalized with respect to heart rate, may provide a valuable index of regional function.

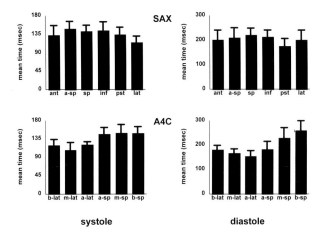

Figure 10.12. Regional mean time of left ventricular ejection (left) and filling (right) obtained from regional fraction area change data (see text) in the short axis (top) and apical four-chamber (bottom) views. Data represents the average of 12 normal subjects, standard deviations are shown for each segment.

Integrated fractional area change time curves obtained in each subject provided a simple display of the temporal progression of ejection and filling phases (Figure 10.13). When combined, these curves reflected changes in LV area throughout the cardiac cycle, including the rapid filling, diastasis and atrial filling phases of diastole. In the short axis view, total systolic and diastolic fractional area changes were 66±6% and 77±7%, respectively. In contrast, in the apical four-chamber view, the corresponding values were 28±6% and 36±8%.

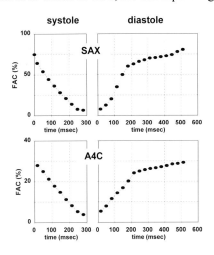

Figure 10.13. Time curves of global fractional area change (FAC), in percent of global left ventricular end-diastolic area, integrated with respect to the time during contraction (left panels) and relaxation (right panels) in the short axis (SAX, top) and apical four-chamber (A4C, bottom) views. Data shown was obtained in one subject.

Regional time curves reflecting integrated area change (Figure 10.14) and integrated radial shortening showed almost identical temporal patterns, which were similar to those reflecting global fractional area change (Figure 10.13). These regional patterns were uniform between segments and consistent between subjects. In most segments, ejection and filling phases (including rapid filling, diastasis and atrial filling) were clearly noted.

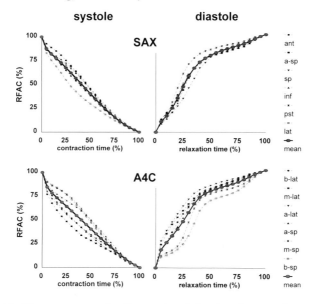

Figure 10.14. Time curves reflecting regional fractional area change (RFAC) integrated with respect to time. To allow inter-segment comparisons, both axes were normalized so that in each segment, fractional area change is 100% at 100% of ejection or filling time. Data represents the average of 12 normal subjects.

Normal Response to Pharmacological Interventions

In order to determine how Color Kinesis images are affected by different pharamacological agents with opposing profiles, 14 normal subjects were studied. The magnitude and temporal patterns of systolic endocardial motion were assessed using intravenous infusions of the β-agonist dobutamine, β-blocker esmolol and atropine.

Dobutamine versus Esmolol

End-systolic Color Kinesis images were initially obtained in 7 normal subjects (age 33±3) under: (1) control conditions; (2) esmolol (200 µg/kg/min); and (3) dobutamine (15 µg/kg/min).

Figure 10.15 (top) shows end-systolic Color Kinesis images obtained from one subject under control conditions, and during infusions of esmolol and dobutamine. In all subjects, consistent differences in color distribution were observed with each pharmacological intervention. With esmolol, the relative contribution of early colors (orange and yellow) was reduced when compared with control conditions, indicating reduced endocardial motion in early systole. In contrast, dobutamine resulted in increased contribution of the early colors, reflecting augmented endocardial motion during early systole.

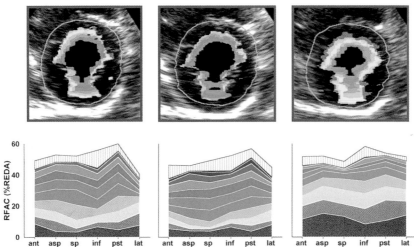

Figure 10.15. Example of end-systolic Color Kinesis images (top) obtained from a normal subject in the short axis view; from left to right: under control conditions, during infusion of esmolol (200 µg/kg/min), and during infusion of dobutamine (15 µg/kg/min). The stacked color histograms of regional fractional area change shown below each image represent the average of 7 normal subjects at the corresponding phase (standard deviations are shown as a dashed band).

These observations were confirmed by quantitative segmental analysis of end-systolic Color Kinesis images. Figure 10.15 (bottom) shows the summary of results dispalyed as stacked color histograms reflecting regional incremental fractional area change in percent of segmental end-diastolic area in the short axis view, under control conditions (left), esmolol (center) and dobutamine (right). Please note the differences in color distribution between the different phases reflecting variations in the temporal patterns of endocardial motion.

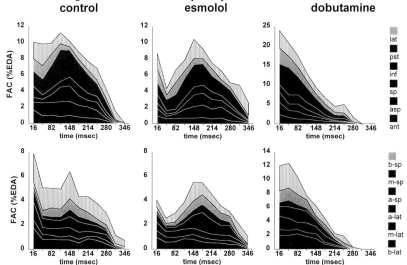

Figure 10.16. Ejection rate as a function of time, in units of LV end-diastolic area (EDA) per second in the short axis (top) and apical four-chamber (bottom) views: under control conditions (left), esmolol (center) and dobutamine (right). Data from different segments is displayed as stacked histograms, and represents the average of 7 normal subjects; standard deviations are shown as a dashed band.

Plots of ejection rate versus time demonstrated the drug-induced differences in overall left ventricular function (Figure 10.16). These differences quantified using indices of global left ventricular function are summarized in Table 10.2. When compared to control conditions, the total area under the time-histogram, reflecting global left ventricular fractional area change, and the magnitude of the histogram peak, reflecting peak ejection rate, decreased with esmolol and increased with dobutamine. Time to peak ejection rate and mean time of contraction were both prolonged with esmolol and shortened with dobutamine, when compared to baseline. The regional mean time of contraction also reflected these pharmacological effects on a regional basis (Figure 10.17).

Table 10.2. Summary of indices of global left ventricular function under control conditions, and under infusions of esmolol and dobutamine: FAC - fractional area change; PER - peak ejection rate; TPER - time to peak ejection rate, and <t> - mean time of contraction, averaged for 12 segments in both short axis (SAX) and apical four-chamber (A4C) views. Data represents the average of 7 normal subjects. Statistical significance of differences when compared with control conditions is shown for each drug (NS - non-significant, p>0.05).

		control	esmolol		dobutamine	
		mean ± sd	mean ± sd	p	mean ± sd	p
HR (bpm)		57 ± 7	54 ± 7	NS	81 ± 7	<0.001
FAC (%EDA)	SAX	67 ± 3	59 ± 5	<0.003	81 ± 6	<0.001
	A4C	31 ± 8	28 ± 4	NS	43 ± 10	<0.03
PER (EDA/sec)	SAX	3.1 ± 0	2.9 ± 0.4	NS	6.1 ± 1	<0.001
	A4C	1.8 ± 1	1.5 ± 0.3	NS	2.9 ± 1	<0.01
TPER (msec)	SAX	115 ± 33	137 ± 59	NS	22 ± 12	<0.001
	A4C	82 ± 66	165 ± 71	<0.05	49 ± 33	NS
<t> (msec)	SAX	132 ± 12	160 ± 11	<0.001	88 ± 13	<0.001
	A4C	137 ± 13	160 ± 12	<0.005	89 ± 11	<0.001

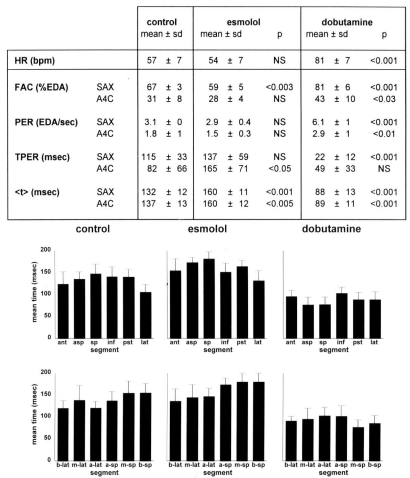

Figure 10.17. Mean time of contraction for each segment in the short axis (top) and apical four-chamber (bottom) views: control (left), esmolol (center) and dobutamine (right). Data represents the average of 7 normal subjects.

Regional time curves also reflected the variations in the temporal progression of regional LV contraction (Figure 10.18). The slope of the initial portion of the curves corresponding to early systole decreased with esmolol and increased with dobutamine. For example, in the short axis view, at 50% time, 61±2% contraction was completed under control conditions, while 54±4% was completed with esmolol (p<0.001), and 78±5% with dobutamine (p<0.001).

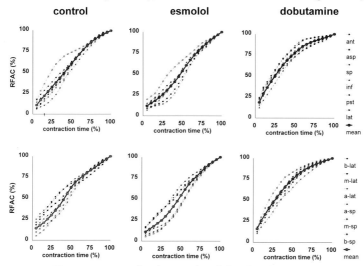

Figure 10.18. Time curves reflecting regional fractional area change (RFAC) integrated with respect to time, in the short axis (top) and apical four-chamber (bottom) views: under control conditions (left), esmolol (center) and dobutamine (right). To allow inter-segment comparisons, both axes were normalized so that in each segment, fractional area change is 100% at 100% of ejection time. Data represents the average of 7 normal subjects.

In this study, segmental analysis of Color Kinesis images provided quantitative evaluation of the temporal patterns of global as well as regional endocardial motion. This technique proved sensitive to depict changes in inotropic state induced by drug inteventions.

Dobutamine versus Atropine

This study was designed to determine the relative contributions of augmented contractility versus increased heart rate towards the variations in Color Kinesis images observed with dobutamine. This protocol was conducted in 7 normal

subjects (age 32±6). Following data acquisition under control conditions, Color
Kinesis images were obtained under three different intravenous infusion doses
of dobutamine (5, 10 and 15 µg/kg/min). After termination of the dobutamine
infusion, when heart rate reached its baseline level, atropine was administered in
increments of 0.2 mg. Data acquisition was repeated when heart rate reached the
level observed with the highest dose of dobutamine.

Figure 10.19 summarizes the dose-dependent effects of dobutamine on the
patterns of systolic endocardial motion observed in the short axis view. When
compared with control conditions (top, left), the relative contribution of early
colors consistently grew with increasing doses of dobutamine (bottom, left to
right), reflecting increased endocardial motion early in systole. Interestingly,
with atropine (top, right), the color distribution of the histogram was similar to
that seen under baseline conditions, despite the differences in heart rate.

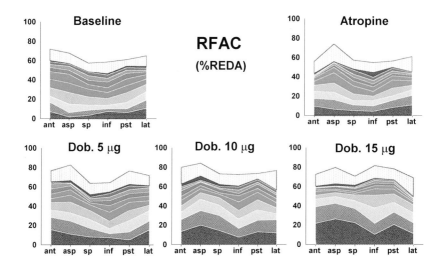

Figure 10.19. Regional incremental fractional area change (RFAC) in percent of
regional end-diastolic area (REDA) in the short axis view under control
conditions (top, left), increasing doses of dobutamine (bottom, left to right), and
atropine (top, right). Color encoding scheme is shown at the bottom, region
notations as in Figure 10.5. Data represent the average of 7 normal subjects;
standard deviations are shown as a dashed band.

Plots of ejection rate versus time also demonstrated gradual dose-dependent variations which are summarized in Table 10.3 in terms of indices of global left ventricular function. Dobutamine resulted in a significant increase in fractional area change and peak ejection rate. Time to peak ejection rate and mean time of contraction shortened consistently under increasing doses of dobutamine. In contrast, with atropine, no significant differences were found in these parameters, when compared to baseline.

Table 10.3. Summary of indices of global LV function under control conditions, with incremental infusions of dobutamine, and with atropine (see Table 10.2 for abbreviations). Data represents the average of 7 normal subjects. Statistical significance of differences when compared with control conditions is shown for each drug (NS = non-significant, p>0.05).

		control	dob. 5		dob. 10		dob. 15		atropine	
		mean ± sd	mean ± sd	p	mean ± sd	p	mean ± sd	p	mean ± sd	p
HR (bpm		64 ± 8	70 ± 7	NS	88 ± 16	<0.005	111 ± 15	<0.001	107 ± 18	<0.001
FAC (%EDA)	SAX	68 ± 10	76 ± 7	NS	87 ± 3	<0.001	89 ± 8	<0.001	70 ± 14	NS
	A4C	35 ± 9	40 ± 5	NS	46 ± 4	<0.05	52 ± 8	<0.003	40 ± 16	NS
PER (EDA/sec)	SAX	3.5 ± 0.6	4.5 ± 1.1	NS	6.3 ± 1.4	<0.001	9.4 ± 3.3	<0.001	4.0 ± 1.3	NS
	A4C	1.6 ± 0.4	2.1 ± 0.6	NS	3.5 ± 1.2	<0.002	4.3 ± 1.4	<0.001	2.1 ± 0.8	NS
TPER (msec)	SAX	126 ± 16	55 ± 35	<0.001	33 ± 17	<0.001	27 ± 16	<0.001	88 ± 52	NS
	A4C	102 ± 61	95 ± 45	NS	36 ± 26	<0.001	29 ± 16	<0.001	82 ± 36	NS
<t> (msec)	SAX	135 ± 8	117 ± 12	<0.01	102 ± 21	<0.002	77 ± 25	<0.001	120 ± 15	<0.05
	A4C	143 ± 17	126 ± 15	NS	103 ± 22	<0.003	99 ± 22	<0.001	133 ± 4	NS

Regional time curves reflected the dobutamine dose-dependent variations in the temporal progression of regional left ventricular contraction (Figure 10.20). When compared with control conditions (top, left), the slope of the initial portion of the curves consistently increased with increasing dose of dobutamine (bottom, left to right), reflecting augmented endocardial motion early in systole. The temporal progression of contraction with atropine (top, right) was similar to that observed at baseline, in spite of significantly different heart rates.

The results of this study showed that the effects of dobutamine on systolic Color Kinesis images are dose dependent. Using atropine, we proved that dobutmine-induced variations in the temporal sequence of endocadial motion as reflected by Color Kinesis, were not significantly affected by the chronotropic effect of the drug, but rather a result of augmented myocardial contractility.

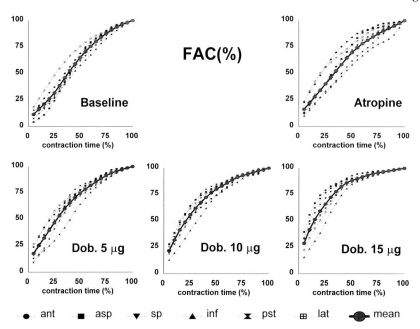

Figure 10.20. Time curves reflecting regional fractional area change (RFAC) integrated with respect to time, obtained in the short axis view: under control conditions (top, left), increasing doses of dobutamine (bottom, left to right), and atropine (top, right). To allow inter-segment comparisons, both axes were normalized so that in each segment, fractional area change is 100% at 100% of ejection time. All data represent the average of 7 normal subjects.

Limitations of Color Kinesis

Color Kinesis was developed to assess endocardial motion, rather than wall thickening. The impact of this limitation on the clinical utility of this technique has yet to be determined. Moreover, similar to acoustic quantification and other techniques, the success of Color Kinesis depends on the quality of echocardiographic images [27,35]. However, in our experience, it is possible to obtain reliable Color Kinesis data in 80 to 85% of consecutive patients.

A limitation which is particularly relevant to quantifying the temporal aspects of endocardial motion is the relatively low temporal resolution imposed by the fixed frame rate of 30 Hz (in NTSC systems) at which Color Kinesis color-encodes pixel transitions. The temporal resolution becomes even lower for imaging systems based on the European standard which operate at 25 Hz. At this relatively low frame rate, Color Kinesis only provides up to 11 sampling points for the entire duration of systolic contraction and 19 points for diastole. The duration of both systole and diastole may shorten with dobutamine, which causes the current temporal resolution to become even more inadequate. This low resolution may not allow sufficient definition of endocardial motion to accurately measure temporal indices of regional left ventricular function.

Accuracy of the timing of color-encoding during both systole and diastole is extremely important for acquisition of Color Kinesis images. For example, at heart rates lower than 55 bpm, color-encoding of the entire diastolic period usually requires more than the currently available nineteen frames. In these cases, the contribution of atrial contraction towards left ventricular filling may be partially missed. Therefore, diastolic Color Kinesis images should be interpreted with caution in patients with very slow heart rates. These limitations could be overcome by using higher frame-rate imaging [47] in conjunction with an extended color scale.

It is also important to remember that the empirical formula used to determine the timing of color-encoding (eq. 1) depends on the presence of a regular rhythm to accurately determine the timing of end-systole on a beat-to-beat basis. Therefore, in patients with irregular rhythms, Color Kinesis data should be acquired and interpreted with special care.

Similar to other methods that quantify endocardial excursion, Color Kinesis is affected by cardiac translation and/or rotation [7,10]. Therefore, if significant translation or rotation is present, as occurs at times in patients with large pericardial effusion or during exercise, Color Kinesis may incorrectly depict endocardial motion, and data should be interpreted with caution. Also, respiration can result in translation artifacts, which can be minimized by acquiring data during held end-expiration. Repeated acquisition strategy combined with averaging may also assure more reliable results.

Limitations of Analysis Techniques

While we have performed quantitative analysis of data obtained in the short axis and apical four-chamber views only, the feasibility and accuracy of this approach in other standard views (parasternal long axis and apical two-chamber views), has yet to be determined. Another limitation of our method is the manual determination of the anatomic landmarks used in the segmentation models, rather than automated identification, which can be extremely difficult. However, in our experience, these landmarks are usually easy to identify, even in patients with suboptimal image quality.

Summary

In this chapter, we have described the principles of operation and technical guidelines for acquisition of a new echocardiographic technique designed to track and display endocardial motion in real time. This technique is based on acoustic quantification but differs from the existing automated border detection in its ability to demonstrate in a single frame both magnitude and timing of regional endocardial motion, providing a basis for objective quantification. Detailed quantitative segmental analysis of Color Kinesis images results in a variety of readily accessible indices of both magnitude and timing of endocardial motion. These indices were investigated in normal subjects both at baseline and under various pharmacological agents known to affect left ventricular function. The following chapter will describe the studies designed to explore the potential clinical utility of these indices for the assessment of regional systolic and diastolic left ventricular performance.

Acknowledgements

We gratefully acknowledge our colleagues at the University of Chicago Noninvasive Cardiac Imaging Laboratories. We wish to acknowledge the valuable contributions of our sonographers: Lynn Weinert, James Bednarz, Claudia Korcarz, Joanne Sandelski and Beth Balasia, who acquired the data for these studies. Without their help and dedication, this project would never have crystallized. We are specially indebted to Rick Koch for his contribution.

References

1.   Lang RM, Vignon P, Weinert L, Bednarz J, Korcarz C, Sandelski J, Koch R, Prater D, Mor-Avi V: Echocardiographic quantification of regional left ventricular wall motion using Color Kinesis. *Circulation* 1996;93:1877-1885

2. Schiller NB, Shah PM, Crawford M, DeMaria A, Devereux R, Feigenbaum H, Gutgessel H, Reichek N, Sahn D, Schnittger I, Silverman NH, Tajik AJ: Recommendations for quantitation of the left ventricle by two-dimensional echocardiography. *J Am Soc Echocardiogr* 1989;2:358-367

3. Pellikka PA, Roger VL, Oh JK, Miller FA, Seward JB, Tajik AJ: Stress Echocardiography. Part II. Dobutamine stress echocardiography: techniques, implementations, clinical applications, and correlations. *Mayo Clinic Proceedings* 1995;70:16-27

4. Topol EJ, Traill TA, Fortuin NJ: Hypertensive hypertrophic cardiomyopathy of the elderly. *N Engl J Med* 1985;312:277-283

5. Bonow RO, Bacharach SL, Green MV, Kent KM, Rosing DR, Lipson LC, Leon MB, Epstein SE: Impaired left ventricular diastolic filling in patients with coronary artery disease: assessment with radionuclide angiography. *Circulation* 1981;64:315-323

6. Appleton CP, Hatle LK, Popp RL: Relation of transmitral flow velocity patterns to left ventricular diastolic function: new insights from a combined hemodynamic and Doppler echocardiographic study. *J Am Coll Cardiol* 1988;12:226-240

7. Shub C, Klein AL, Zachariah PK, Bailey KR, Tajik AJ: Determination of left ventricular mass by echocardiography in a normal population: effect of age and sex in addition to body size. *Mayo Clin Proc* 1994;69:205-211

8. Klein AL, Burstow DJ, Tajik AJ, Zachariah PK, Bailey KR, Seward JB: Effects of age on left ventricular dimensions and filling dynamics in 117 normal persons. *Mayo Clin Proc* 1994;69:212-224

9. Bahl VK, Dave T, Sundaram KR, Shrivastava S: Pulsed Doppler echocardiographic indices of left ventricular diastolic function in normal subjects. *Clin Cardiol* 1992;15:504-512

10. Friedman BJ, Drinkovic N, Miles H, Shih WJ, Mazzoleni A, DeMaria AN: Assessment of left ventricular diastolic function: comparison of Doppler echocardiography and gated blood pool scintigraphy. *J Am Coll Cardiol* 1986;8:1348-1354

11. Spirito P, Maron BJ, Bonow RO: Noninvasive assessment of left ventricular diastolic function: comparative analysis of Doppler echocardiographic and radionuclide angiographic techniques. *J Am Coll Cardiol* 1986;7:518-526

12. Chenzbraun A, Pinto FJ, Popylisen S, Schnittger I, Popp RL: Filling patterns in left ventricular hypertrophy: a combined acoustic quantification and Doppler study. *J Am Coll Cardiol* 1994;23:1179-1185

13. Samstad SO, Torp HG, Linker DT, Rossvoll O, Skjaerpe T, Johansen E, Kristoffersen K, Angelsen BAJ, Hatle L: Cross sectional early mitral flow velocity profiles from colour Doppler. *Br Heart J* 1989;62:177-184

14. Bryg RJ, Williams GA, Labovitz AJ: Effect of aging on left ventricular diastolic filling in normal subjects. *Am J Cardiol* 1987;59:971-974

15. Fisher DC, Sahn DJ, Friedman MJ, Larson D, Valdes-Cruz LM, Horowitz S, Goldberg SJ, Allen HD: The mitral valve orifice method for noninvasive two-

dimensional echo Doppler determinations of cardiac output. *Circulation* 1983;67:872-877

16. Ormiston JA, Shah PM, Tei C, Wong M: Size and motion of the mitral valve annulus in man. I. A two-dimensional echocardiographic method and findings in normal subjects. *Circulation* 1981;64:113-120

17. Stoddard MF, Keedy DL, Longaker RA: Two-dimensional transesophageal echocardiographic characterization of ventricular filling in real time by acoustic quantification: comparison with pulsed Doppler echocardiography. *J Am Soc Echo* 1994;7:116-131

18. Brutsaert DL, Rademakers FE, Sys SU: Triple control of relaxation: implications in cardiac disease. *Circulation* 1984;1:190-196

19. Gaasch WH, Blaustein AS, Bing OHL: Asynchronous relaxation of the left ventricle. *J Am Coll Cardiol* 1985;5:891-897

20. Hui WKK, Gibson DG: Mechanisms of reduced left ventricular filling rate in coronary artery disease. *Br Heart J* 1983;50:362-371

21. Aoyagi T, Pouleur H, Van Eyll C, Rousseau MF, Mirsky I: Wall motion asynchrony is a major determinant of impaired left ventricular filling in patients with healed myocardial infarction. *Am J Cardiol* 1993;72:268-272

22. Bonow RO, Vitale DF, Bacharach SL, Frederick TM, Kent KM, Green MV: Asynchronous left ventricular regional function and impaired global diastolic filling in patients with coronary artery disease: reversal after coronary angioplasty. *Circulation* 1985;71:297-307

23. Bonow RO, Vitale DF, Maron BJ, Bacharach SL, Frederick TM, Green MV: Regional left ventricular asynchrony and impaired global left ventricular filling in hypertrophic cardiomyopathy: effect of verapamil. *J Am Coll Cardiol* 1987;9:1108-1116

24. St.John Sutton MG, Tajik AJ, Gibson DG, Brown DJ, Seward JB, Giulliani ER: Echocardiographic assessment of left ventricular filling and septal and posterior wall dynamics in idiopathic hypertrophic subaortic stenosis. *Circulation* 1978;57:512-520

25. Kumada T, Karliner JS, Pouleur H, Gallagher KP, Shirato K, Ross J: Effects of coronary occlusion on early ventricular diastolic events in conscious dogs. *Am J Physiol* 1979;237:H542-H549

26. Yamagishi T, Ozaki M, Kumada T, Ikezono T, Shimizu T, Furutani Y, Yamaoka H, Ogawa H, Matsuzaki M, Matsuda Y, Arima A, Kusukawa R: Asynchronous left ventricular diastolic filling in patients with isolated disease of the left anterior descending coronary artery: assessment with radionuclide ventriculography. *Circulation* 1984;69:933-942

27. Kondo H, Masuyama T, Ishihara K, Mano T, Yamamoto K, Naito J, Nagano R, Kishimoto S, Tanouchi J, Hori M, Takeda H, Inoue M, Kamada T: Digital subtraction high-frame-rate echocardiography in detecting delayed onset of regional left ventricular relaxation in ischemic heart disease. *Circulation* 1995;91:304-312

11 Clinical Applications of Color Kinesis: Facts Versus Hopes

Victor Mor-Avi, Philippe Vignon
and Roberto M. Lang

Color Kinesis is a new echocardiographic technique based on acoustic quantification that tracks endocardial motion by color-encoding pixel transitions between blood and myocardial tissue in real time. Color Kinesis generates an integrated display of magnitude and timing of endocardial motion in a single end-systolic or end-diastolic frame, which provides the basis for objective evaluation of regional myocardial performance. In the previous chapter we described the principles of operation of this new technology and the technical guidelines for data acquisition. We also reviewed the methods of segmental analysis of Color Kinesis images which have been developed to allow the quantification of both the magnitude and timing of left ventricular endocardial motion during both systolic ejection and diastolic filling.

The present chapter will present the potential clinical applications of Color Kinesis. First, we will describe how this method can be used for objective detection of regional wall motion abnormalities at rest and during dobutamine stress testing [1]. Thereafter, we will describe how myocardial ischemia affects the normal temporal sequences of endocardial motion. In the second part of this chapter, we will describe the use Color Kinesis as a tool to assess global as well as regional diastolic function.

Automated Detection of Regional Wall Motion Abnormalities

In order to test the feasibility of objective detection of regional systolic wall motion abnormalities, we acquired Color Kinesis images in 20 normal subjects (mean age: 49±18 years) and in 40 patients with regional wall motion abnormalities diagnosed by two-dimensional echocardiography (mean age: 66 ± 13 years). Exclusion criteria were: (1) inadequate image quality; (2) pericardial effusion, (3) rhythm disturbances, (4) abnormal interventricular septal motion due to previous sternotomy, right ventricular pressure or volume overload, and/or left bundle branch block, (5) inability to track wall motion with acoustic quantification in over 30% of the endocardial boundary.

Histograms of incremental LV fractional area change obtained in the normal subjects were averaged to obtain the normal pattern of endocardial motion. These average histograms were then used as a normal reference for comparison with those obtained from patients with suspected regional wall motion abnormalities. To facilitate objective detection of regional wall motion abnormalities, individual histograms obtained from each patient were superimposed on the normal reference defined as one standard deviation around the mean of the normal control group. Regional wall motion abnormalities were diagnosed when the regional fractional area change in at least one segment deviated from this normal reference.

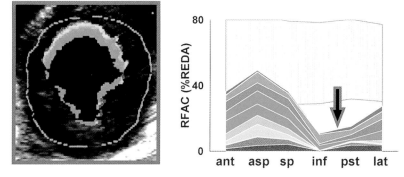

Figure 11.1. Example of an end-systolic Color Kinesis image obtained in a patient with regional wall motion abnormality (left). To allow objective diagnosis, a histogram of regional fractional area change (RFAC) was superimposed on the corresponding normal reference (dashed band). The gap between the normal reference and the individual data reflects hypokinesis in the inferior, posterior and lateral segments (arrow). REDA - regional end-diastolic area.

Figures 11.1 and 11.2 show examples of data obtained from patients with regional wall motion abnormalities. These Figures present the end-systolic color-encoded images with the corresponding individual histograms superimposed on the averaged normal reference to allow objective detection of regional wall motion abnormalities. In the example shown in Figure 11.1, the gap between the normal values and the individual patient's data demonstrates areas of hypokinesis in the inferior, posterior and lateral segments. The deviation from the normal range in these specific segments can be detected automatically (see arrow). Similarly, Figure 11.2 demonstrates hypokinesis in the anteroseptal and inferoseptal segments in the short axis view as well as apical- and mid-septal segments in the apical four-chamber view.

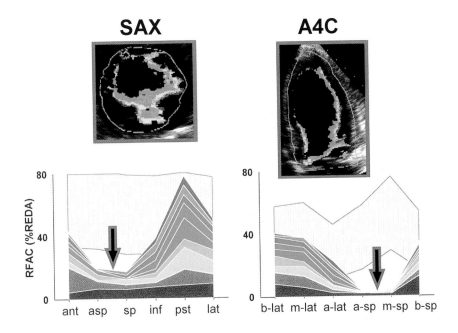

Figure 11.2. Example of Color Kinesis data obtained in a patient with regional wall motion abnormalities (see legend to Figure 11.1 for details). The gaps between the normal reference and the individual data in both the short axis (left) and apical four-chamber (right) views reflect the hypokinesis noted in the mid-anteroseptal and mid-inferoseptal regions, as well as mid- and apical septal segments (arrows). Modified with permission from the American Heart Association, *Circulation* 1996; 93:1877–1888.

Figure 11.3 shows an example of Color Kinesis images obtained in a patient with global LV systolic dysfunction secondary to dilated cardiomyopathy. Although the pattern of regional contraction in this case is preserved, the entire histogram is shifted down below the normal reference (lower panels), indicating diffuse systolic dysfunction.

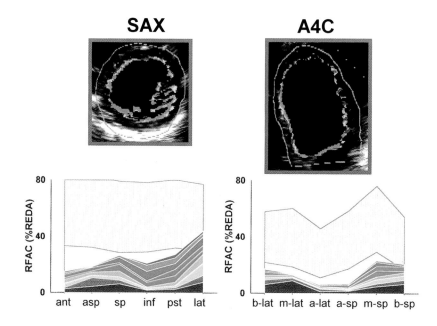

Figure 11.3. Example of Color Kinesis data and results of segmental analysis that demonstrate global hypokinesis in a patient with dilated cardiomyopathy. Note the global deviation from the normal pattern of contraction in the apical four-chamber view.

To evaluate the feasibility of automated detection of regional wall motion abnormalities, the following protocol was conducted. Initially, videotapes of two-dimensional echo-cardiographic short axis and apical four-chamber views obtained from 40 patients with regional wall motion abnormalities were independently reviewed by two experienced readers. Regional wall motion abnormalities were identified using a conventional segmentation scheme [2]. The diagnostic variability between readers was calculated as the number of discordant interpretations divided by the total number of segments defined as abnormal by at least one of the two readers. Subsequently, in order to reach consensus, discordant segments were reviewed jointly by both readers. Finally, to obtain data on the inter-technique variability, the consensus interpretation was compared with the results of the automated detection of regional wall motion abnormalities on a region-by-region basis.

The inter-observer variability in the interpretation of regional systolic wall motion based on visual inspection of two-dimensional echocardiograms was 13.5% (divergence in 31 of 230 segments diagnosed as abnormal by at least one observer). The inter-technique variability between the consensus reading and the automated method, was found to be 17.0% (divergence in 35 of 206 segments diagnosed as abnormal by the consensus reading). This inter-technique variability was not significantly different from the inter-observer variability of the conventional interpretation. In other words, in this group of patients, segmental analysis of Color Kinesis images allowed automated detection of regional wall motion abnormalities, which was found to be as accurate as that provided by experts interpreting two-dimensional echocardiograms.

Regional Wall Motion During Dobutamine Stress Testing

To test the feasibility of using segmental analysis of Color Kinesis images for objective evaluation of regional wall motion during dobutamine stress echocardiography, images were obtained in 20 patients (mean age: 62±2 years). A standard protocol for dobutamine stress testing [3] was followed. Images were acquired at baseline, low and peak dobutamine infusion rates, and during recovery. At each phase, Color Kinesis was activated to color-encode systolic endocardial motion. Image sequences with Color Kinesis overlays were saved in digital format on optical disks for subsequent off-line analysis.

Initially, visual interpretation of two-dimensional images was performed by an experienced reader of dobutamine stress echocardiograms who reviewed the digitally stored loops of two-dimensional images without Color Kinesis overlays displayed. In each view, the comparisons between different phases of the protocol were performed using a side-by-side display in a quad-screen format. The interpretation was based in each view on segmentation schemes recommended by the American Society of Echocardiography [2]. In each patient, regional endocardial motion was examined visually, and judged as either normal or abnormal response to dobutamine.

Subsequently, end-systolic Color Kinesis images were subjected to the above described computer analysis of regional wall motion. Dobutamine induced regional wall motion abnormalities were defined as segments that displayed >40% reduction in regional fractional area change with dobutamine relative to baseline values. This threshold for automated detection was set based on the previously described normal variability of up to 20% in Color Kinesis data obtained under resting conditions [1]. This automated detection of dobutamine induced regional wall motion abnormalities was compared on a segment by segment basis to the conventional visual interpretation. Statistics of agreement and disagreement between methods were obtained in terms of under- and overscoring by the automated detection method.

Figure 11.4 shows an example of end-systolic short axis images with Color Kinesis overlays obtained in a patient who had a normal response to dobutamine. The gradual increase in the colored area with increasing doses of dobutamine reflects the positive inotropic effects of the drug, which resulted in LV cavity obliteration at peak infusion rate. In addition, the progressively growing contribution of orange and yellow colors reflects the uniform increase in LV endocardial motion during early systole, similar to that noted in normal subjects (see Figures 10.15 and 10.19).

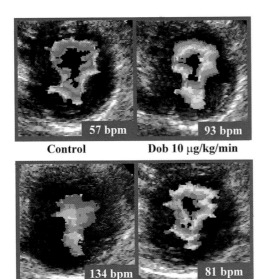

57 bpm

93 bpm

Control   **Dob 10 μg/kg/min**

134 bpm

81 bpm

Dob 40 μg/kg/min   **Recovery**

Figure 11.4. Example of short axis view end-systolic Color Kinesis images obtained in a patient undergoing dobutamine stress testing (images correspond to 4 consecutive phases of a standard stress protocol; heart rates are shown). Please note the prevalence of orange and yellow colors reflecting increased endo-cardial excursion during early systole.

Figure 11.5 presents an example of data obtained in a patient who developed a significant wall motion abnormality during dobutamine infusion. This figure displays stacked histograms of regional incremental fractional area change calculated from the apical four-chamber view under control conditions (left), low dose (center) and peak dose (right). Histograms obtained with dobutamine are superimposed on that obtained under control conditions (shown as a dashed band on the background) to allow objective detection of dobutamine induced regional wall motion abnormalities. While endocardial motion of the lateral wall augmented with dobutamine, the septal wall developed mild hypokinesis at low dose and became severely hypokinetic to akinetic at high dose (see arrows).

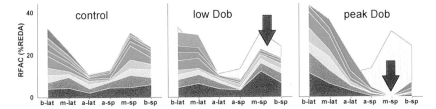

Figure 11.5. Stacked histograms of regional fractional area change obtained from apical four-chamber end-systolic Color Kinesis images in a patient undergoing dobutamine stress testing: under control conditions (left), low dose (center) and peak dose (right). Histograms obtained with dobutamine were superimposed on that obtained under control conditions shown as a dashed band on the background. Please note the progressive appearance of hypokinesis in the septal wall with increasing dose of dobutamine (arrows).

Visual interpretation of two-dimensional images obtained during pharmacological stress testing detected dobutamine induced regional wall motion abnormalities in 10 out of 20 patients (38 of 360 segments examined). Segmental analysis of end-systolic Color Kinesis images detected reduced endocardial motion as compared to control conditions in 36 out of these 38 segments (95%). The two cases of apparent failure to detect regional wall motion abnormalities (5%) were found to be the result of discordance between the visual interpretation of segment size and automated analysis of end-systolic Color Kinesis images. In addition, segmental analysis of Color Kinesis showed reduced fractional area change in 5 out of other 322 segments classified as normal during conventional visual interpretation (<2%). These false positive interpretations were the result of inadequate endocardial tracking, confirmed by repeated examination of image sequences with and without Color Kinesis.

In order to determine the clinical value of this methodology, as well as its sensitivity and specificity, these initial findings need to be confirmed in a larger population of consecutive patients referred for dobutamine stress echocardiography. However, it is clear that this technique is easy and objective, and therefore may prove as a useful adjunct to conventional visual interpretation of two-dimensional images acquired during dobutamine stress testing.

Temporal Heterogeneity of Left Ventricular Systole

The following study was performed in order to determine whether segmental analysis of Color Kinesis images can identify regional abnormalities in the temporal sequence of systolic endocardial motion. We calculated the mean time of contraction for each myocardial segment in the above described population of 40 patients with baseline regional wall motion abnormalities. This parameter was displayed as a bar diagram (Figure 10.12). In each patient, the mean time of

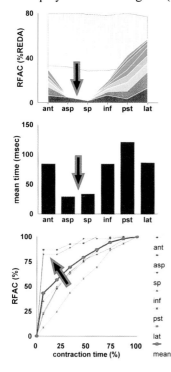

contraction was averaged separately for normal and abnormal segments. The ratio of the abnormal to normal segments was then calculated and averaged for the entire group. In most segments identified as abnormal, the mean time of contraction was shorter when compared to normal segments (Figure 11.6, top and middle). The mean time of contraction ratio between the abnormal and normal segments was 0.78±0.21.

Figure 11.6. Data obtained in a patient with severe hypokinesis of the anteroseptal and septal segments. The hypokinesis is reflected in the histogram of regional fractional area change (top) by the gap between the normal range and the individual data (arrow). The mean time of contraction (middle) regions is markedly shortened as in these specific compared with other segments (arrow). The regional time curves obtained from the hypokinetic segments reveal that 80% of the motion in these segments occurred within the first 33 msec of systole (bottom, arrow).

The regional time curves depicting the temporal progression of LV ejection had steeper initial slopes compared to segments with normal endocardial motion (Figure 11.6, bottom). These findings indicate that the residual motion in abnormal segments occurs early in systole.

These observations were subsequently confirmed during dobutamine stress testing. Figure 11.7 shows an example of data obtained in a patient who developed a regional wall motion abnormality during dobutamine infusion. At baseline, regional fractional area change (top, left) as well as the mean time of ejection (bottom, left) were normal. With a low dose of dobutamine, the septal segments developed mild hypokinesis relative to baseline (top, center). Interestingly, the mean time of ejection in these segments did not change, whereas in the lateral wall which augmented appropriately, the mean time shortened compared to baseline (bottom, center). At peak dobutamine, the mid- and basal-septal segments became severely hypokinetic (top, right). The mean time of ejection in these segments shortened compared to other segments, which augmented appropriately in response to dobutamine (bottom, right).

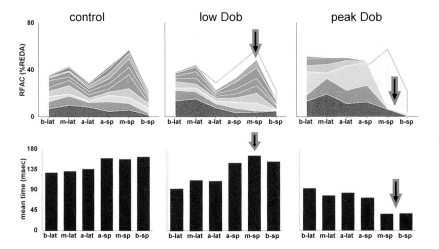

Figure 11.7. Example of data obtained in a patient undergoing dobutamine stress testing. With low dose, the septal segments showed magnitude of motion slightly below the baseline level (top, center). The mean time of ejection in these segments did not change, whereas in the lateral wall, the mean time was short compared to baseline (bottom, center). At peak dose, mid- and basal-septal segments became severely hypokinetic (top, right). The mean time of ejection in these segments shortened compared with other segments (bottom, right).

These observations suggest that myocardial ischemia may cause delayed endocardial motion in mildly hypokinetic segments. In contrast, the residual motion in severely hypokinetic segments occurs early in systole. This biphasic effect of ischemia on the temporal sequence of systolic contraction has yet to be confirmed in future animal studies, where regional myocardial ischemia can be induced by gradual coronary ligations and alterations in the temporal sequence of endocardial motion tracked under controlled conditions. The assessment of temporal aspects of systolic endocardial motion on a regional basis could potentially increase the sensitivity of dobutamine stress testing and offer additional insight into the mechanisms involved in wall motion abnormalities.

Assessment of Global Left Ventricular Diastolic Function

Abnormalities in LV diastolic filling often precede the development of systolic dysfunction in various disease states such as cardiac hypertrophy [4] and coronary artery disease [5]. Left ventricular diastolic properties are commonly evaluated indirectly by noninvasively measuring transmitral blood flow velocities with pulsed-Doppler ultrasound. However, the diagnosis of diastolic dysfunction in patients with normalized flow velocity patterns [6] remains a challenging problem.

To determine the clinical value of Color Kinesis images for the evaluation of global LV diastolic function, Doppler and Color Kinesis data were compared between patients with left ventricular hypertrophy (LVH) and age-matched controls. Accordingly, 25 patients (age: 55 ± 14 years) with concentric LVH (LV mass index 178 ± 52 g/m^2) secondary to long-standing systemic hypertension were enrolled. Exclusion criteria were: (1) pericardial effusion and previous pericardotomy; (2) arrhythmias and conduction abnormalities; (3) heart rates below 55 or above 100 beats per minute; (4) moderate to severe mitral or aortic regurgitation assessed with color-flow Doppler; (5) mitral or aortic valve stenosis; and (6) dynamic LV outflow tract obstruction. The control group consisted of 25 age-matched normal subjects (age: 54 ± 14 years; LV mass index 67 ± 14 g/m^2) selected based on the following inclusion criteria: (1) normal two-dimensional echocardiogram; (2) mitral flow velocity pattern (E/A ratio and deceleration time) normalized for age and gender [7-9]; (3) absence of valvular heart disease. All subjects enrolled had normal LV systolic function without evidence of regional wall motion abnormalities. No significant differences in heart rate were noted between hypertensive patients and normal subjects.

Patients were divided into two groups based on their Doppler mitral inflow patterns by comparing the individual E/A ratios and deceleration times with the previously reported 95% confidence intervals, obtained in a normal population over a wide range of ages [8,9]. Group 1 included 12 patients with an abnormal relaxation pattern characterized by reduced E/A ratios and prolonged deceleration times. Group 2 included 13 patients with age and gender normalized E/A ratios: 7 patients with prolonged and 6 with normal deceleration times. In each group, Color Kinesis data were compared with conventional Doppler-derived indices. In addition, Color Kinesis and Doppler data were compared between groups and corresponding age-matched controls.

In all study subjects, a complete transthoracic echocardiographic study including M-mode, two-dimensional imaging, pulsed wave Doppler and color flow mapping of valvular orifices was performed, as well as diastolic Color Kinesis image acquisition. Isovolumic relaxation time was measured as the time interval between the aortic valve closure click and the onset of the mitral valve inflow. Peak velocities during rapid filling (E) and atrial contraction (A) as well as the area under each peak velocity (VTI_E and VTI_A) were measured. Subsequently, the early to late diastolic mitral flow velocity ratio (E/A ratio) and the ratio of the areas under both the E and A waves were calculated. In addition, the deceleration time was also measured. Pulmonary vein inflow velocities were measured at end-expiration and the ratio between peak forward flow velocity during ventricular systole and diastole (S/D ratio) was calculated.

Table 11.1. Pulsed wave Doppler-derived indices obtained in two groups of patients with concentric LV hypertrophy and in age-matched controls.

Group	N	IRT (msec)	E/A ratio	VTI_E /VTI_A	DT (msec)	S/D ratio
Abnormal relaxation (Group 1)	12	122 ± 34*	0.73 ± 0.18*	1.46 ± 0.39*	316 ± 108*	1.67 ± 0.42*
Controls	12	75 ± 11	1.26 ± 0.32	2.01 ± 0.42	199 ± 34	1.32 ± 0.35
Normalized mitral inflow (Group 2)	13	100 ± 24*	1.21 ± 0.46	2.00 ± 0.88	235 ± 58	1.19 ± 0.40
Controls	13	74 ± 12	1.20 ± 0.27	1.81 ± 0.44	192 ± 21	1.26 ± 0.31

*: $p \leq 0.05$ when compared with controls. *Abbreviations*: IRT = isovolumic relaxation time; E/A = ratio between the peak velocities of early (E wave) and late (A wave) diastolic mitral inflow; VTI = velocity time integral; DT deceleration time; S/D = ratio between the peak velocities of forward pulmonary vein flow during systole (S wave) and diastole (D wave).

Mitral and pulmonary venous flow Doppler-derived indices obtained in the two groups of patients with LVH and corresponding controls are shown in Table 11.1. When compared to the respective controls, the isovolumic relaxation time was prolonged in all patients with LVH. The pulmonary vein S/D ratio was augmented in group 1, but similar to controls in patients with normalized mitral flow Doppler patterns (Table 11.1, group 2).

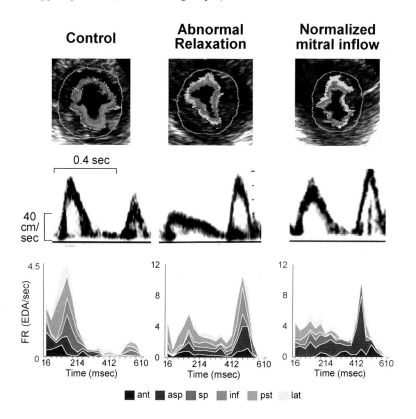

Figure 11.8. Examples of end-diastolic Color Kinesis images (top) with the corresponding time-histograms of filling rate, FR, (bottom) obtained in three subjects with distinct transmitral Doppler flow profiles (middle). When compared to the normal subject (left), the time-histogram of the patient with abnormal relaxation (middle) exhibited predominant late diastolic colors, resulting in an inverted Peak1/Peak2 ratio reflecting a markedly increased contribution of atrial contraction towards LV filling. Please note that the patient with normalized mitral inflow Doppler profile (right) had a similar Color Kinesis pattern.

Figure 11.8 shows examples of end-diastolic Color Kinesis images obtained in two patients with LVH and an age-matched control subject. Despite similar heart rates, the hypertensive patients exhibited increased endocardial displacement late in diastole compared to the control subject, reflecting the augmented contribution of atrial contraction towards LV filling [10-12]. These findings were objectively confirmed by the time-histograms of filling rate (bottom) which were similar to the respective mitral inflow Doppler profiles (middle) in normal subjects and in group 1 patients.

Table 11.2. Color Kinesis parameters of global LV diastolic function obtained in the two groups of patients with cardiac hypertrophy and in corresponding age-matched normal subjects. *: $p \leq 0.05$ when compared with controls; SAX - short axis view, A4C - apical four-chamber view.

Group	N	Peak1 / Peak2 ratio		Mean time of filling (msec)	
		SAX	A4C	SAX	A4C
Abnormal relaxation (Group 1)	12	1.67 ± 0.74*	1.57 ± 0.53	255 ± 33*	225 ± 21*
Controls	12	3.48 ± 1.74	2.31 ± 1.86	198 ± 22	193 ± 19
Normalized mitral inflow (Group 2)	13	1.86 ± 1.03*	1.71 ± 1.05*	236 ± 34	226 ± 35*
Controls	13	3.20 ± 1.70	2.49 ± 0.71	227 ± 31	201 ± 24

The time-histograms had two distinct peaks: one occurring early in diastole corresponding to rapid LV filling, and the second occurring late in diastole, reflecting the contribution of atrial contraction towards LV filling. The Peak1/Peak2 ratio was diminished in patients with abnormal relaxation and correlated closely with the VTI_E/VTI_A ratio (r=0.78; $p<0.001$). In addition, the mean LV filling time was prolonged in group 1 patients (Table 11.2). Similar to group 1 patients, the time-histograms obtained in group 2 exhibited a disproportionately large contribution of atrial contraction towards LV filling compared to controls despite the presence of normalized mitral Doppler flow velocity tracings (Figure 11.9). Accordingly, Peak1/Peak 2 ratio was reduced and mean LV filling time prolonged in patients with normalized mitral flow (Table 11.2). As a result, in these patients, VTI_E/VTI_A correlated poorly with Peak1/Peak2 obtained from Color Kinesis time-histograms (r=0.44; p=0.02).

Thus, in patients with either abnormal relaxation or normalized mitral flow Doppler profiles, Color Kinesis time-histograms depicted a reduced contribution of rapid LV filling compensated by augmented atrial contraction. Since time-histograms paralleled mitral flow Doppler profiles in group 1, the relative contributions of rapid filling and atrial contraction towards LV filling assessed with both techniques correlated closely. Accordingly, in patients with abnormal relaxation, the instantaneous transmitral blood flow velocities driven by the pressure gradient between left atrium and ventricle appeared to directly reflect instantaneous volumetric LV filling. However, Color Kinesis time-histograms and mean LV filling time were abnormal in group 2 patients, whereas Doppler indices were similar to those obtained in age-matched controls.

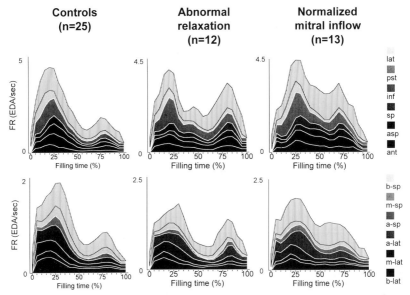

Figure 11.9. Averaged time-histograms displaying the temporal profile' of diastolic filling rate (FR) in normal subjects (left) and in two groups of patients with LVH, obtained from Color Kinesis images in the short axis (top) and apical four-chamber (bottom) views. The dashed band represents the standard deviation of the mean. Increased fractional area change during late diastole, consistent with augmented atrial contribution towards LV filling, is evident in both group 1 (abnormal relaxation) and group 2 (normalized mitral inflow).

This discrepancy between instantaneous variations in LV inflow velocities and diastolic fractional area change can be explained by the following reasons. First, studies have recently shown that the mitral flow velocity does not have a flat spatial profile as initially assumed [13]. Second, blood flow entering the left ventricle appears to be oriented differently in early versus late diastole [14].

Third, the mitral annulus cross-sectional area has been shown not only to gradually increase as diastole progresses [14-16], but also to change in shape [16]. Finally, the mitral inflow is three-dimensional whereas pulsed-Doppler measurements are performed at a single location of a two-dimensional plane.

Therefore, quantitative analysis of end-diastolic Color Kinesis images allows fast and objective evaluation of global LV diastolic function, sensitive enough to identify diastolic dysfunction in patients presenting with normalized mitral inflow Doppler profiles. As such, this method may also prove clinically useful in identifying global diastolic dysfunction in various disease states.

Assessment of Regional Diastolic Properties

Methods used for serial assessment of LV diastolic function such as Doppler echocardiography and acoustic quantification provide information on global rather than regional LV filling [12,17]. Global LV diastolic function is adversely influenced by heterogeneities in both the timing and magnitude of regional contraction and relaxation [18,19]. To fully understand this relationship, regional diastolic properties need to be elucidated in normal subjects and in patients with heart disease. Diagnostic techniques currently available to assess regional LV diastolic performance, such as contrast or nuclear ventriculography [20-23], require injection of contrast or radio-pharmaceutical substances and extensive off-line data processing. We studied the ability of segmental analysis of Color Kinesis images to objectively assess regional LV diastolic properties by quantifying the timing and magnitude of diastolic endocardial motion. In particular, our study was designed to determine whether quantitative segmental analysis of end-diastolic Color Kinesis images can objectively characterize regional diastolic LV wall motion asynchrony.

We studied temporal indices of regional diastolic endocardial motion derived from end-diastolic Color Kinesis images obtained in a group of 25 patients with concentric LVH and a control group of 25 age-matched normotensive subjects. In normal subjects, the patterns of LV endocardial motion were consistent and relatively uniform, as demonstrated by the homogeneous regional time-curves (Figure 11.10, top). In contrast, patients with concentric LVH frequently exhibited diastolic endocardial motion asynchrony (Figure 11.10, middle). This asynchrony was also corroborated by the presence of wide intersegmental variability in the regional mean LV filling times (Figure 11.10, bottom).

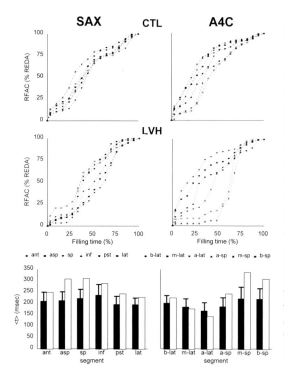

Figure 11.10. Examples of regional time curves obtained in a normal subject (top) and a patient with LVH (middle). In the normal subject, the curves are uniform in both the short axis (SAX) and apical four-chamber (A4C) views. Tthe patient with LVH exhibited diastolic endocardial motion asynchrony, reflected by inhomogeneous regional filling curves (middle) and mean filling times (<t>; bottom). Bar histograms show regional mean LV filling times obtained in this patient (open bars) compared with average values of 29 normal subjects (solid bars).

Regional time-curves obtained in normal subjects were averaged. In each segment, a reference pattern of endocardial diastolic motion was defined as one standard deviation around the mean and used for objective diagnosis of regional diastolic dysfunction. Figure 11.11 shows an example of regional LV filling curves obtained in a patient with LVH and normal LV systolic function, superimposed on the corresponding reference profiles. In this patient, regional diastolic endocardial motion was clearly delayed in the anterior, anteroseptal and septal segments, as reflected by the downward shift of these curves relative to the corresponding reference profiles. As a result, the mean regional LV filling time was consistently prolonged (Figure 11.11).

The percentage of total endocardial motion completed at 50% of the LV filling period was computed for each segment from the integrated regional time-curves, and averaged for all segments. The standard deviation of the mean was used to objectively reflect regional diastolic wall motion heterogeneities occurring during the rapid LV filling period in each subject. Individual standard deviations were compared between patients with LVH and age-matched controls. In patients with LVH, the proportion of total diastolic regional fractional area change completed during the first half of the LV filling period was significantly reduced when compared with age-matched controls (64±10% vs. 75±7%, *p*<0.001). When compared to controls, regional diastolic endocardial motion was more heterogeneous in hypertensive patients, as reflected by the larger standard deviations around the mean regional fractional area change at 50% of LV filling period (10.9 vs. 7.7%: *p*=0.001). These findings are in agreement with previous studies [23,24], where increased diastolic wall motion nonuniformity has been reported in association with impaired global LV relaxation in patients with cardiac hypertrophy.

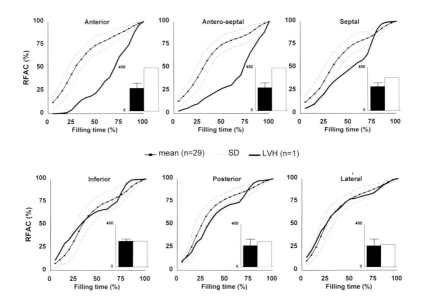

Figure 11.11. Example of regional normalized filling curves obtained in a patient with concentric LVH and normal systolic function. For each segment, a reference profile of diastolic endocardial motion was generated by averaging curves obtained in 29 normal subjects; the dashed lines represent one standard deviation around the mean. In this case, the individual curves in the anterior, anteroseptal and septal segments were shifted downwards relative to the reference profile, reflecting delayed endocardial motion during early diastole. For each segment, the mean time of filling (<t> in msec) is displayed (open bars) together with the mean normal values (solid bars) for comparison.

Physiologic nonuniformity in regional diastolic endocardial motion appears to be present in the normal heart to maintain LV diastolic performance within an optimal range of mechanical efficiency by modulating ventricular relaxation [18]. Assuming that overall LV diastolic function is no more than the sum of its regional diastolic properties, one might suggest that an inappropriate increase in diastolic wall motion nonuniformity may result in uncoordinated and consequently prolonged LV relaxation in patients with concentric hypertrophy. However, Bonow et al. [23] reported that a small group of patients (15%) with cardiac hypertrophy and preserved systolic function exhibited homogeneous regional LV filling when evaluated using radionuclide angiography. Similarly, in our study, 12% of patients with LV hypertrophy and preserved systolic performance had no evidence of diastolic endocardial motion asynchrony.

Importantly, it has been demonstrated in multiple experimental and clinical studies that diastolic wall motion asynchrony constitutes a major mechanism responsible for impaired LV relaxation in ischemic heart disease [21,22,25,26]. By providing an objective tool to detect delayed diastolic endocardial motion, analysis of Color Kinesis images has the potential of identifying regional diastolic dysfunction, which in the ischemic cascade, appears to occur before systolic wall motion abnormalities become evident [22,26,27].

Summary

In this chapter, we described our initial clinical experience with Color Kinesis. We believe that this new technology has significant clinical potential which stems directly from its intrinsic properties. Color Kinesis images may become a useful aid for the evaluation of regional endocardial wall motion by less experienced readers of echocardiograms, as Color Kinesis display directs the physician's attention towards specific hypokinetic segments. This technique may also become helpful in conveying echocardiographic findings to referring physicians because a single end-systolic or end-diastolic image contains the entire sequence of systolic or diastolic endocardial motion and has the advantage of easy digital storage and retrieval. Furthermore, segmental analysis of Color Kinesis images provides objective automated detection of regional wall motion abnormalities manifested as variations in either magnitude or timing of regional endocardial wall motion in systole and diastole. This ability has the potential to improve the sensitivity of echocardiographic stress testing and possibly aid in the assessment of myocardial viability.

References

1. Lang R, Vignon P, Weinert L, Bednarz J, Korcarz C, Sandelski J, Koch R, Prater D, Mor-Avi V: Echocardiographic quantification of regional left ventricular wall motion using Color Kinesis. *Circulation* 1996;93:1877-1885.
2. Schiller NB, Shah PM, Crawford M, DeMaria A, Devereux R, Feigenbaum H, Gutgessel H, Reichek N, Sahn D, Schnittger I, Silverman NH, Tajik AJ: Recommendations for quantitation of the left ventricle by two-dimensional echocardiography. *J Am Soc Echocardiogr* 1989;2:358-367.
3. Pellikka PA, Roger VL, Oh JK, Miller FA, Seward JB, Tajik AJ: Stress Echocardiography. Part II. Dobutamine stress echocardiography: techniques, implementations, clinical applications, and correlations. *Mayo Clinic Proceedings* 1995;70:16-27.
4. Topol EJ, Traill TA, Fortuin NJ: Hypertensive hypertrophic cardiomyopathy of the elderly. *N Engl J Med* 1985;312:277-283.
5. Bonow RO, Bacharach SL, Green MV, Kent KM, Rosing DR, Lipson LC, Leon MB, Epstein SE: Impaired left ventricular diastolic filling in patients with coronary artery disease: assessment with radionuclide angiography. *Circulation* 1981;64:315-323.
6. Appleton CP, Hatle LK, Popp RL: Relation of transmitral flow velocity patterns to left ventricular diastolic function: new insights from a combined hemodynamic and Doppler echocardiographic study. *J Am Coll Cardiol* 1988;12:226-240.
7. Shub C, Klein AL, Zachariah PK, Bailey KR, Tajik AJ: Determination of left ventricular mass by echocardiography in a normal population: effect of age and sex in addition to body size. *Mayo Clin Proc* 1994;69:205-211.
8. Klein AL, Burstow DJ, Tajik AJ, Zachariah PK, Bailey KR, Seward JB: Effects of age on left ventricular dimensions and filling dynamics in 117 normal persons. *Mayo Clin Proc* 1994;69:212-224.
9. Bahl VK, Dave T, Sundaram KR, Shrivastava S: Pulsed Doppler echocardiographic indices of left ventricular diastolic function in normal subjects. *Clin Cardiol* 1992;15:504-512.
10. Friedman BJ, Drinkovic N, Miles H, Shih WJ, Mazzoleni A, DeMaria AN: Assessment of left ventricular diastolic function: comparison of Doppler echocardiography and gated blood pool scintigraphy. *J Am Coll Cardiol* 1986;8:1348-1354.
11. Spirito P, Maron BJ, Bonow RO: Noninvasive assessment of left ventricular diastolic function: comparative analysis of Doppler echocardiographic and radionuclide angiographic techniques. *J Am Coll Cardiol* 1986;7:518-526.
12. Chenzbraun A, Pinto FJ, Popylisen S, Schnittger I, Popp RL: Filling patterns in left ventricular hypertrophy: a combined acoustic quantification and Doppler study. *J Am Coll Cardiol* 1994;23:1179-1185.
13. Samstad SO, Torp HG, Linker DT, Rossvoll O, Skjaerpe T, Johansen E, Kristoffersen K, Angelsen BAJ, Hatle L: Cross sectional earlhy mitral flow velocity profiles from colour Doppler. *Br Heart J* 1989;62:177-184.

14. Bryg RJ, Williams GA, Labovitz AJ: Effect of aging on left ventricular diastolic filling in normal subjects. *Am J Cardiol* 1987;59:971-974.

15. Fisher DC, Sahn DJ, Friedman MJ, Larson D, Valdes-Cruz LM, Horowitz S, Goldberg SJ, Allen HD: The mitral valve orifice method for noninvasive two-dimensional echo Doppler determinations of cardiac output. *Circulation* 1983;67:872-877.

16. Ormiston JA, Shah PM, Tei C, Wong M: Size and motion of the mitral valve annulus in man. I. A two-dimensional echocardiographic method and findings in normal subjects. *Circulation* 1981;64:113-120.

17. Stoddard MF, Keedy DL, Longaker RA: Two-dimensional transesophageal echocardiographic characterization of ventricular filling in real time by acoustic quantification: comparison with pulsed Doppler echocardiography. *J Am Soc Echo* 1994;7:116-131.

18. Brutsaert DL, Rademakers FE, Sys SU: Triple control of relaxation: implications in cardiac disease. *Circulation* 1984;1:190-196.

19. Gaasch WH, Blaustein AS, Bing OHL: Asynchronous (segmental early) relaxation of the left ventricle. *J Am Coll Cardiol* 1985;5:891-897.

20. Hui WKK, Gibson DG: Mechanisms of reduced left ventricular filling rate in coronary artery disease. *Br Heart J* 1983;50:362-371.

21. Aoyagi T, Pouleur H, Van Eyll C, Rousseau MF, Mirsky I: Wall motion asynchrony is a major determinant of impaired left ventricular filling in patients with healed myocardial infarction. *Am J Cardiol* 1993;72:268-272.

22. Bonow RO, Vitale DF, Bacharach SL, Frederick TM, Kent KM, Green MV: Asynchronous left ventricular regional function and impaired global diastolic filling in patients with coronary artery disease: reversal after coronary angioplasty. *Circulation* 1985;71:297-307.

23. Bonow RO, Vitale DF, Maron BJ, Bacharach SL, Frederick TM, Green MV: Regional left ventricular asynchrony and impaired global filling in hypertrophic cardiomyopathy: effect of verapamil. *J Am Coll Cardiol* 1987;9:1108-1116.

24. St.John Sutton MG, Tajik AJ, Gibson DG, Brown DJ, Seward JB, Giulliani ER: Echocardiographic assessment of left ventricular filling and septal and posterior wall dynamics in hypertrophic subaortic stenosis. *Circulation* 1978;57:512-520.

25. Kumada T, Karliner JS, Pouleur H, Gallagher KP, Shirato K, Ross J: Effects of coronary occlusion on early ventricular diastolic events in conscious dogs. *Am J Physiol* 1979;237:H542-H549.

26. Yamagishi T, Ozaki M, Kumada T, Ikezono T, Shimizu T, Furutani Y, Yamaoka H, Ogawa H, Matsuzaki M, Matsuda Y, Arima A, Kusukawa R: Asynchronous left ventricular diastolic filling in patients with isolated disease of the left anterior descending coronary artery: assessment with radionuclide ventriculography. *Circulation* 1984;69:933-942.

27. Kondo H, Masuyama T, Ishihara K, Mano T, Yamamoto K, Naito J, Nagano R, Kishimoto S, Tanouchi J, Hori M, Takeda H, Inoue M, Kamada T: Digital subtraction high-frame-rate echocardiography in detecting delayed onset of regional left ventricular relaxation in ischemic heart disease. *Circulation* 1995;91:304-312.

12 Doppler Myocardial Imaging

George R. Sutherland, Aleksandra Lange, Przamyslaw Palka, Norma McDicken

Current standard cardiac ultrasound techniques derive their information on myocardial function indirectly based either on parameters measured from the endo- and epicardial specular reflections or from blood pool Doppler indices.

Doppler Myocardial Imaging (DMI) is a new cardiac ultrasound technique in which Doppler signal processing is applied to the reflected ultrasound signals originating within the myocardium [1,2]. Information on myocardial function can be derived from the use of either color Doppler principles or by performing either spectral or power analysis of the pulsed Doppler signal derived from a sample volume placed within the myocardium. In the color Doppler approach, mean velocity estimation is based on the autocorrelation technique and quantifies regional intramural velocities by detecting consecutive phase shifts of the reflected echoes from myocardium. The use of Doppler techniques to interrogate myocardial motion is not a new concept. Pulsed Doppler recordings of myocardial motion using a single sample volume technique were first described by Isaaz *et al.* in 1989 [3]. Although deemed to be interesting, little clinical value was ascribed at that time to this approach. It was not until 1991 that McDicken *et al.* [4] first described the modifications required to a standard cardiac ultrasound system which would allow visualization of the motion of a tissue-equivalent phantom that the potential clinical value of color Doppler processing of myocardial signals began to be appreciated.

Doppler signal processing of myocardial ultrasound information has several theoretical advantages over standard gray scale imaging. Doppler processing has an intrinsically lower noise floor and a higher signal to clutter ratio. Doppler processing allows the accurate measurement of differing mean myocardial velocities at a large number of neighboring intra-mural sites. (This is inherently simpler, quicker and more reliable than the alternative technique of tracking the speckle pattern within conventional B and M-Mode images). In addition, as both spectral and color Doppler techniques measure frequency shift rather than signal amplitude, any velocity image information thus obtained is less affected by tissue attenuation than gray scale imaging. (Thus, it is frequently possible to obtain diagnostic image quality DMI images from patients who appear "poorly echogenic" on standard gray scale imaging). Where gray scale imaging remains superior to color Doppler imaging is in its inherent higher spatial resolution and (in current generation equipment) higher frame rates. Yet despite both current frame rate and resolution limitations, the color Doppler technique can provide clinical diagnostic information. Current generation ultrasound processing techniques allied to digital signal processing within the new generation of ultrasound machines allow color Doppler images to be displayed with a frame rate of 50-80/second. While image spatial resolution is inferior to gray scale imaging, this approaches 1 x 1 mm at low color Doppler frame rates and 2 x 2 mm at frame rates of 40-50/sec.

Doppler Myocardial Imaging: Technical Considerations

In a conventional ultrasound machine, prior to blood pool Doppler signal processing taking place, the reflected Doppler ultrasound signal is passed through a high-pass (clutter) filter which will reject the high intensity, low-frequency components arising from the myocardium. Thus to visualize the myocardium, an ultrasound machine must be adapted. This is effected by changing the thresholding and filtering algorithms to reject the low amplitude echoes from the blood pool and to allow the high amplitude, low velocity information from the myocardium to pass to subsequent determination of the mean Doppler shift, and hence mean velocity, using standard autocorrelation methodology (Figure 12.1).

The mean velocity information thus derived may be displayed in either a two-dimensional (Figure 12.2) or M-Mode format. From the mean velocity information, the machine can also be programmed to calculate and display regional myocardial accelerations in a two-dimensional format (although with a reduced frame rate). In addition, a further myocardial Doppler parameter can be measured and displayed - the power of the Doppler signal (Figure 12.3).

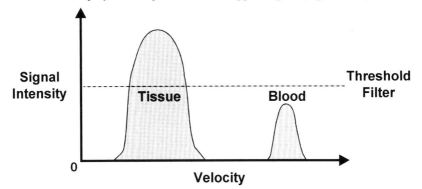

Figure 12.1. This figure illustrates the principles underlying the implementation of Doppler Myocardial Imaging. To obtain tissue information as opposed to blood pool Doppler information, the signal intensity threshold filter has to be altered. In addition, algorithms have to be changed to allow encoding of the low velocities at which the myocardium moves with concomitant rejection of high velocity blood pool information.

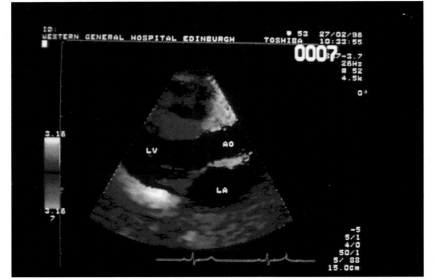

Figure 12.2. A left ventricular long axis Doppler myocardial image. Note that within the posterior wall, a gradation of velocities is seen with the highest recorded sub-endocardially and the lowest sub-epicardially.

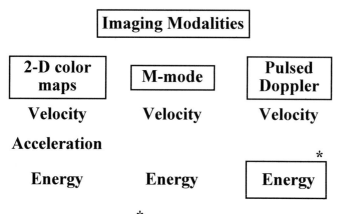

Figure 12.3. This figure lists the currently available formats in which Doppler myocardial imaging information can be obtained. (Note that the M-Mode of acceleration is simply velocity information and thus an M-Mode of acceleration data is not available).

Doppler Myocardial Imaging: *In Vitro* Studies

A series of *in vitro* phantom studies [5] have confirmed the accuracy of DMI velocity encoding over the range of velocities at which normal and abnormal myocardium would be expected to move (Figure 12.4). Velocity estimation has been shown to be affected by target velocity, target material, system receive gain and the pulse train size but the inherent error is at worst ± 10% of the true mean velocity [5]. The spatial resolution of both the two-dimensional velocity and power maps is at best 1 x 1 mm and at worst 3 x 3 mm with a slightly inferior axial resolution compared to standard gray-scale imaging but a similar lateral resolution [2]. This means that the DMI technique is a better real-time spatial discriminator than real time MRI, Position Emission Tomography or current nuclear perfusion techniques.

Doppler Power (Energy) Interrogation of the Myocardium

The power (or signal strength) of reflected myocardial Doppler ultrasound information is directly related to the number of scatterers within the tissue block exposed to ultrosound. Thus, measurement of regional Doppler power levels could provide information on tissue characterization. The Doppler power signal is both velocity independent and angle independent as this measurement is independent of the phase-shift of the signal. Regional Doppler power can be displayed in two formats: as a two-dimensional image (currently with a dynamic range of 0-40 dB) or as the temporal variation in signal strength of the signal derived from a pulsed Doppler sample volume placed within the myocardium (but excluding the endocardial and pericardial specular reflectors). This latter measurement can be obtained by measuring the power of the raw audio data (which is available on all ultrasound machines) using a specially developed on-line power meter. The temporal variations in power levels can then be fed back into the machine via an auxiliary channel and displayed as a trace in real time simultaneously with the Doppler myocardial velocity information. Raw audio data is relatively unprocessed ultrasound information obtained early in the signal processing path with the ultrasound machine; it has a wide dynamic range (typically 0-70 dB) and is linearly processed data. This should be the direct equivalent of integrated backscatter data derived from the myocardium. Using a similar Doppler power measurement technique, Schwartz *et al.* [6] have already demonstrated in a series of *in vitro* studies that single pulsed Doppler power measurement is the direct equivalent of integrated backscatter measurement in terms of changes in blood pool reflectivity produced by varying the concentrations of an echo contrast agent.

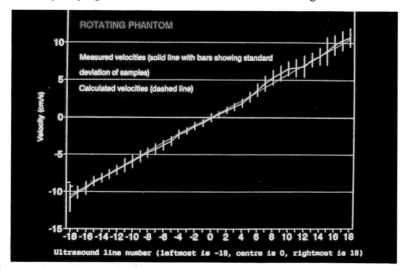

Figure 12.4: The result of an *in vitro* study in a tissue equivalent phantom in which predicted mean velocitiy is plotted against measured mean velocity.

DMI Studies of Normal Myocardial Function:
Circumferential Contractile Function

To circumvent the temporal resolution problems inherent in the first generation of DMI systems in determining intra-mural velocities using the two dimensional approach, DMI M-Mode interrogation of intramural velocities was developed. This technique allows myocardial sampling at approximately 4 millisecond intervals with high spatial resolution but as with all M-Mode techniques should only be carried out where insonnating the myocardium at 90°. Such M-Mode velocity studies in normal patients have confirmed the presence of transmural systolic and diastolic velocity gradients across the left and right ventricular walls during the cardiac cycle (Figure 12.3) [7,8,9,10]. These velocity gradients are presumed to represent circumferential contractile function only and are in accord with prior reports on intramural velocity gradients recorded by placement of a series of ultrasonic crystals within the myocardium during animal experiments. These latter studies have also recorded an early systolic transmural velocity gradient with higher velocities encoded in the sub-endocardial region and lowest velocities in the sub-epicardial region. A series of DMI M-Mode velocity studies have confirmed the normal velocity distribution and timing of peak velocity gradients within the left ventricular posterior wall and inter-ventricular septum during the cardiac cycle. These studies have also identified predictable changes in intramural velocities which occur associated with aging.

Longitudinal Contractile Function

DMI M-Mode studies have also been used to interrogate long-axis shortening of the heart by aligning the M-Mode beam along the apex-base axis of the inter-ventricular septum or lateral left and right ventricular walls. These studies have demonstrated a base-to-apex longitudinal velocity gradient in both the septum and ventricular free walls with the highest long-axis shortening velocities recorded at the cardiac base and with almost zero velocities recorded at the apex (Figure 12.5).

Thus the DMI technique has the potential to characterize long-axis function of the heart including regional abnormalities in long-axis contraction and relaxation. With respect to both circumferential and longitudinal contractile function, DMI velocities have also been shown to change in a predictable manner in response to both positive and negative inotropic stimulation in an animal model. In addition, single pulsed Doppler DMI velocity sample volume interrogation of the myocardium allows the determination of regional myocardial peak velocities and their temporal relationship to regional mechanical and electrical events in the heart (Figure 12.6).

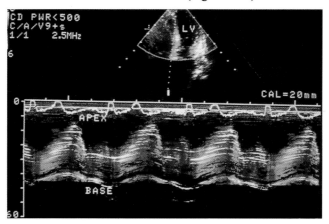

Figure 12.5. A precordial 4-chamber Doppler myocardial image (upper panel) with the M-Mode beam aligned through the ventricular septum in the apex to base orientation. Note the highest contractile and relaxation velocities are recorded towards the base of the heart with virtually no long axis contractile or relaxation velocities present at the apex.

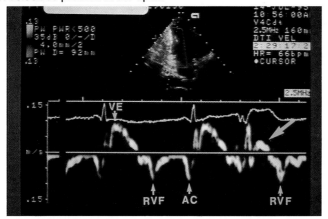

Figure 12.6. A pulsed Doppler myocardial imaging study in a normal patient. The image is acquired from the apical 2-chamber view with a sample volume placed in the inferior wall. The first beat recorded is in normal sinus rhythm with the third beat being a ventricular premature beat. Note the changes in long axis systolic function induced by the premature beat.

Left Ventricular Diastolic and Left Atrial Function

Current ultrasound parameters used to evaluate LV diastolic function are indirect indices derived either from digitized M-Mode traces of the endocardial surfaces or from Doppler indices derived from blood flow through the left heart. DMI provides a direct measure of intramural velocities during LV relaxation and hence may provide a better and more clinically relevant measure of diastolic function. Early studies have shown that DMI indices parallel transmitral Doppler blood flow measurements and normal changes in these latter indices associated with aging [9]. Other studies have shown that measured DMI diastolic velocities of long axis lengthening to correlate with atrio-ventricular valve ring velocities during diastole [11,12]. In addition, DMI indices have been shown to correlate well with both left atrial wall function indices and indices of left atrial appendage function [13,14]. To what extent these new indices provide more clinically relevant information remains to be determined, but it is likely that such direct measurements may supplant current indirect measurements of left ventricular diastolic function.

DMI Studies in Cardiomyopathies and Transplant Patients

A series of comparative clinical studies in patients with dilated cardiomyopathies, hypertrophic cardiomyopathies and concentric LV hypertrophy have determined a range of abnormalities in intramural velocities which could not be predicted from either standard gray-scale two dimensional or M-Mode studies. The results of these studies showed a significant decrease in mean velocities and velocity gradients during all systolic phases in patients with dilated cardiomyopathy [15]. In hypertrophic cardiomyopathy patients, velocity gradients were significantly decreased or reversed in all systolic cardiac phases despite apparently normal M-Mode fractional thickening indices [16]. These abnormalities are likely to be due to the abnormal myocardial architecture in patients with hypertrophic cardiomyopathy and may prove to be a new ultrasound marker specific for this condition. Similar studies in patients with infiltrative cardiomyopathies have demonstrated both Doppler velocity and reflectivity changes which seem to mirror the degree of myocardial involvement not always apparent on the gray-scale image. In transplant patients, similar changes in myocardial reflectivity have been shown to correlate well with biopsy-proven early moderate rejection but whether these changes are sufficiently sensitive indicators to be used in routine clinical practice remains to be proven. In addition, pulsed wave Doppler can be used to determine the relative contractile function of both donor and recipient atria.

DMI Studies in Ischemic Heart Disease

It has been clearly demonstrated in both animal models and in patients that both color and spectral DMI can determine a series of predictable changes in myocardial contractile function induced by ischemia [17,18]. The earliest ischemia-induced changes have been recorded using the DMI pulsed Doppler technique to identify regional velocity changes. In a dog model, significant early changes in regional diastolic velocities in the ischemia zone were found after only 15 sec of ischemia while diastolic velocities remained normal in the non-ischemic territories [19]. Later changes in systolic peak velocities were also observed which paralleled changes in the transmural velocity gradient obtained by two dimensional DMI reduction in wall thickening on M-Mode images. Encouraging results have also been reported with regard to reversible ischemic changes detected using the DMI single sample volume pulsed Doppler technique with low-dose dobutamine infusions (Figure 12.7) [20].

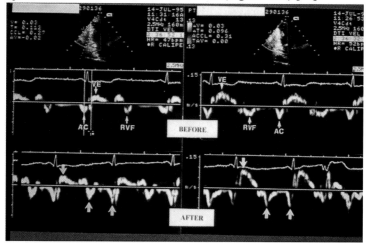

Figure 12.7. Images taken during a low dose dobutamine study for myocardial viability during early and post myocardial infarction. In the upper left panel, the pulsed Doppler sample volume is placed in the apical portion of the inferior LV wall. The apparent double abnormal low velocity contraction pattern seen in systole here is pathognomonic of established infarction. In the lower left panel, during low dose dobutamine, there is no significant change in this myocardial segment during systole but there is an increase in diastolic filling velocities. In the upper right panel, an area which appeared equally contractile in two-dimensional images is shown to be hypo contractile (long axis contractility) prior to low dose dobutamine but function returns to near normal values (lower right) following 5 μg/kg/min of dobutamine. This clearly is viable myocardium.

In areas where infarction has occurred, pulsed Doppler DMI studies of long-axis contractile function would appear to identify a specific and predictive bi-phasic pattern of low velocity myocardial systolic motion which is readily distinguished from the low velocity mono-phasic pattern induced by ischemia in viable myocardium. In addition, predictable changes in transmural velocities associated with a marked reduction in Doppler power signal strength have also been noted in patients with both acute ischemia and infarction (Figure 12.8).

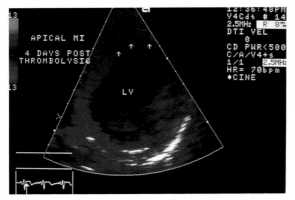

Figure 12.8(A). A short axis view of the LV just below papillary muscle level. The arrows show the area of anterior myocardial infarction. In the subsequent panels, the pulsed Doppler sample volume is tracked around the myocardium from the normally functioning segments, through the peri-infarct ischemic zone and into the infarct.

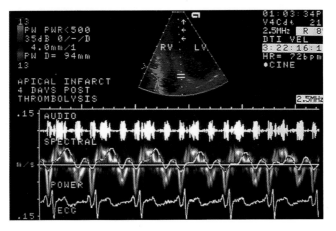

Figure 12.8(B). The normal basal zone.

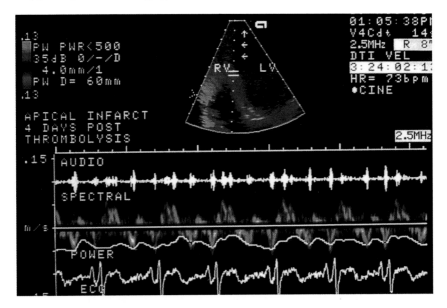

Figure 12.8(C). The peri-infarct ischemic zone.

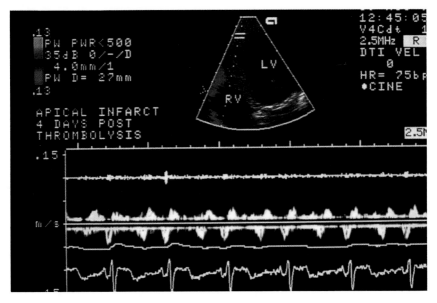

Figure 12.8(D). The infarct zone.

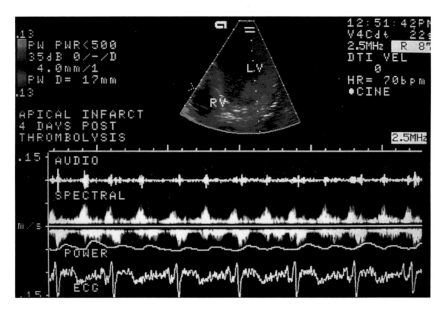

Figure 12.8(E). The viable lateral wall.

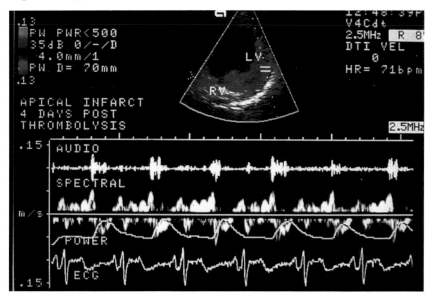

Figure 12.8(F). The normally functioning basal wall.

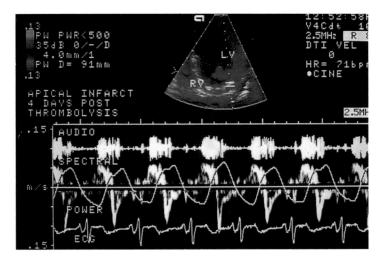

Figure 12.8(G). The amplitude of the power signal is seen to blunt as the infarct area is approached with a flat response in the infarct zone and a return to normal in the lateral wall as tissue viability becomes normal. This paralleled the changes recorded in integrated backscatter levels.

Pulsed Doppler Signal Strength: A Direct Equivalent to Integrated Backscatter Measurements?

Normal and Ischemic Studies

Measurement of variation in the power of the pulsed Doppler myocardial signal from normally contracting myocardium have demonstrated a cyclic variation in signal strength which parallels the temporal variation in standard integrated backscatter measurements. The largest variation in myocardial pulsed Doppler signal strength and highest signal intensities are recorded at the base of the heart with the lowest levels recorded at the apex. These findings again parallel integrated backscatter parameters. Clinical studies have also demonstrated that ischemia blunts both the absolute peak signal levels and the cyclic variation of power of the myocardial pulsed Doppler signal (Figure 12.8). In infarct zones, there is no measurable cyclic variation in pulsed Doppler signal strength although the absolute level of the signal may vary depending on the relative amounts of edema or fibrosis present in the infarct zone. Furthermore, the intensity of the pulsed Doppler myocardial signal can be increased by the presence of a myocardial contrast agent.

DMI Stress Echocardiography: Could This be Feasible?

One initial hope was that, with the appropriate development, Doppler Myocardial Imaging would allow quantification of two dimensional stress echo images by determining ischemia induced intramural velocity changes. The initial low frame rates present in the first generation of DMI two-dimensional imaging systems made such measurements unlikely to be of clinical value. Even with the development of a second generation of DMI instruments with frame rates equal to or greater than current standard 2D gray-scale imaging, the problems associated with the Doppler angle of insonnation of the myocardium continue to preclude off-line measurement of absolute velocity change during stress echo studies. However, subsequent initial DMI studies during low and high dose dobutamine stress echocardiography using the left parasternal window approach have demonstrated a predictable dose dependent increase in mean systolic velocities in both the inferior and anterior left ventricular walls in normal patient while patients with coronary artery disease were shown to have impaired augmentation of systolic velocities [21].

Doppler Power (Energy) Evaluation of Myocardial Perfusion

Current opinion would suggest that the successful detection of regional myocardial perfusion by cardiac ultrasound requires the combination of an effective left heart contrast agent and an appropriate ultrasound detection technique. Gray-scale videodensitometric analysis is increasingly being shown to be inappropriate for myocardial contrast detection due to the inherent gray-scale processing and compression algorithms within the current generation of ultrasound machines. Radiofrequency data acquisition, second harmonic imaging and Doppler power (energy) data acquisition are all more appropriate imaging modalities because of their individual unique properties and linear processing algorithms. Doppler power has been shown to be effective in detecting the presence of a galactose-based left heart contrast agent within the myocardium both in a closed-chest animal model and in normal subjects (Figure 12.9) [2]. Two-dimensional Doppler power imaging has also been shown to detect regional perfusion abnormalities, perfusion changes caused by concomitant dipyridamole infusion and myocardial reperfusion in an animal model [22]. Why should the Doppler power mode offer advantages over gray-scale imaging? Firstly, the mode of ultrasound transmission is different. Doppler power is based on information derived from color Doppler signal processing. To produce an image, the transducer is programmed to send out up to six impulses per line and then waits to receive the returning impulses for a longer period than for a corresponding gray-scale image. This has the effect of delivering more acoustic power to the contrast agent and in a more intermittent manner than gray-scale imaging. As acoustic power is important in creating a non-linear response in contrast agent reflectivity, this may account in part for the greater sensitivity of Doppler power mode imaging. Another factor, which may be important, is the intrinsically lower noise floor of the color Doppler system. It is thus possible that any signal enhancement brought about by the contrast agent may not be identified as it lies within the noise flow of gray-scale imaging but that the same level of signal enhancement would be detected by the Doppler system as it lies above the noise floor. What role any of the Doppler power modalities might play in a clinically effective ultrasound technique remains to be determined but currently it shows equal promise when compared to either radiofrequency data or second harmonic imaging and has a major advantage in its relative ease of implementation within an ultrasound system.

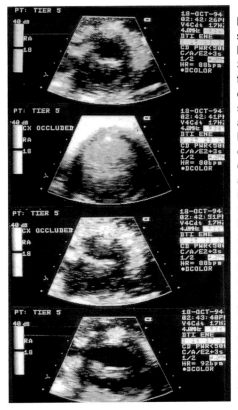

Figure 12.9. A Doppler energy study in an animal model using a left heart contrast agent (Levovist: Schering AG). In the upper panel, the resting LV short axis Doppler energy image is visualized. The second panel shows the contrast agent entering the right and left heart. In the third panel during acute circumflex occlusion, an increase in echo intensity in the normal anterior and lateral zone is seen where no increase is seen in the circumflex (posterior LV wall) territory. In the bottom panel, the clip has been released on the circumflex coronary artery and immediately a return in signal intensity is seen as reperfusion occurs within this wall. It is clear from this series of images that Doppler energy can identify the presence of a left heart contrast agent in a transthoracic animal model and can determine an absolute lack of perfusion and re-perfusion.

DMI Evaluation of Arrhythmias

As DMI can identify regional myocardial velocities and regional variations in myocardial acceleration, theoretically both normal and abnormal patterns of myocardial velocities and accelerations could be identified on a two-dimensional image as could the presence and precise location of foci of onset of abnormal ventricular contraction [23]. In addition, the higher temporal resolution of pulsed Doppler myocardial imaging could also be used to derive instantaneous regional myocardial contraction and relaxation velocities [24]. The normal right and left ventricular myocardial velocity and acceleration sequences during the cardiac cycle have been determined by DMI (2D, pulsed and Doppler and M-Mode) modalities. This data has been compared with myocardial velocity and acceleration information from patients with abnormal ventricular depolarization including patients with pacemakers and bundle branch block. In addition, patients with ventricular arrhythmias and patients with functioning accessory bypass tracts have been studied. The combination of DMI velocity and acceleration mapping using 2D, M-Mode and pulsed DMI techniques can identify specific normal and abnormal sequences of myocardial acceleration which accurately reflected the mode and timing of electrical depolarization. Abnormal early regional changes in velocity or acceleration associated with either Wolff-Parkinson-White bypass tracts, unifocal ventricular premature beats, or sustained ventricular tachycardias have been accurately located as have the immediate normalization in depolarization induced during the monitoring of radiofrequency ablation (Figure 12.10) [24]. This information was only in part available from standard gray-scale imaging. Thus, DMI would appear to be an important new adjunct to the non-invasive investigation of abnormal myocardial depolarization including the real-time monitoring of radiofrequency ablation.

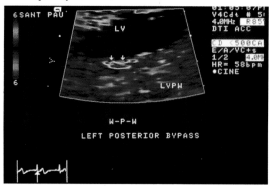

Figure 12.10. A late diastolic frame in a patient with a left-sided Wolff-Parkinson-White bypass tract. The localized early onset of activation (arrowed) of the myocardium is clearly seen in the LV posterior wall situated in a sub-endocardial position.

Doppler Myocardial Imaging: 3D Reconstruction

Three dimensional echocardiography (3DE) is gaining increasing interest as a potentially superior technique to standard 2D echocardiography in the assessment of both congenital and acquired heart disease. To date, 3DE has been applied in the clinical setting in the assessment of (1) left and right ventricular function and volumes, (2) septal defects and (3) native and prosthetic atrio-ventricular valves. Previous studies on 3D reconstruction have used either transesophageal or transthoracic standard gray-scale imaging (GSI) as their data source. A major limitation of the transthoracic approach is the poor quality of the images acquired in a substantial proportion of patients. This is because the quality of GSI image is mainly related to only one parameter, *i.e.* the amplitude of the ultrasound signal returning from the interrogated myocardium which, in a substantial number of patients, is markedly attenuated by the chest wall. The Doppler technique could be used as an alternative tissue-data acquisition technique to overcome problems with low signal to noise ratio. This is due to the fact that, in contrast to GSI imaging, the quality of DMI images is dependent on two factors rather than one: the amplitude of the returning signal (which is in turn, directly dependent on the attenuation) and the frequency shift of this signal which is relatively independent of the attenuation factor. Thus, it is this latter factor which gives rise to the potential of the Doppler technique to provide more complete images of the myocardium than the standard GSI technique [25].

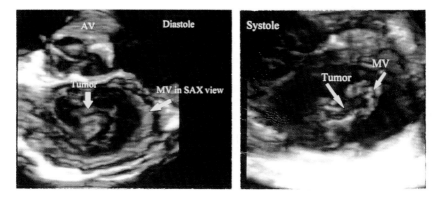

Figure 12.11. A 3D DMI reconstruction of an SLE mass obstructing the mitral valve orifice. The apical short-axis view is the selected reference cut-plane beyond which the system displays all the structures in 3D. Left: with the mitral valve in a closed position, and right: with the mitral valve in an open position as seen from the LV apex.

The first clinical case of 3D DMI reconstruction reported (Figure 12.11) was a unique case of an SLE mass causing acute mitral valve obstruction and mimicking mitral stenosis [26]. Three dimensional DMI information proved to be superior to that obtained from the 3D GSI. Thus, in this case, standard 2D transesophageal images proved unnecessary because the DMI images obtained non-invasively from the precordial approach were of excellent quality, emphasizing the advantage of this technique. These images allowed both the correct quantification of mass volume and determination of its morphology.

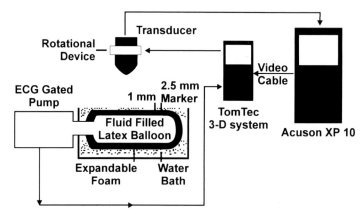

Figure 12.12. The set-up of the *in vitro* study to determine the accuracy and definition of 3D Doppler data acquisition. In order to mimic left ventricle contraction, the phantom was connected to the electrocardiogram gated water pump and de-gassed water was pumped into the phantom at a rate 50 times/min. Specially constructed valve between the phantom and the pump allowed the water from the phantom chamber to be returned back to the pump. to validate the accuracy of the changes in volume measurements, by both techniques GSI and DMI, with changes in size of the measured volume, varying known amounts of water were pumped into the phantom (from 24 ml to 190 ml). In addition, in order to define the minimum size of an isolated reflector which could be accurately identified in a three-dimensional reconstruction by this system, rings of resin crystals of known differing dimension were implanted on the surface of the scanned phantom.

To validate the 3D DMI technique and to assess the potential clinical application of DMI a series of *in vitro* and *in vivo* studies were subsequently performed. To determine the accuracy of 3D DMI imaging both a computer-generated virtual reality phantom and a dynamic tissue-mimicking phantom (Figure 12.12) were used. The aims of these studies were to determine: (1) the minimum size of an isolated crystal which could be determined and the minimum gap which could be seen in the 3D image between 2 separate crystals and (2) the accuracy of 3D volume computation. The analysis of 3D images obtained from the virtual phantom showed that the 3D system could reconstruct structures of 0.3 mm size and identify a gap of 1 mm. Three dimensional images of the tissue-mimicking phantom showed that a crystal of 1 mm could still be seen in both 3D GSI and DMI images. The minimum gap between 2 crystals which could be determined as 1.5 mm for GSI in the central part of the image and 2-3 mm in the peripheral part of the image (Figure 12.13). For DMI, the values were 2 mm and 3 mm, respectively. Both 3D techniques underestimated the true volume of the phantom but the systematic error was smaller for DMI than for GSI over the range of different size of true volume. This study has shown that, although the spatial resolution of the 3D images was virtually identical for both GSI and DMI, DMI is potentially a more accurate acquisition technique in volume measurements. In vivo GSI and DMI 3D LV volume measurements were performed in a group of sixteen patients and the results were correlated with those obtained from biplane cineventriculography [25,26,27]. In vivo, for gray-scale the end-diastolic volume mean difference was -12.6 ml and the limits of agreement were ±18 ml and for DMI the corresponding values were -4.2 and ±10.6 ml, respectively. The difference for end-systole was, for gray-scale -6.5±10.6 ml and for the Doppler technique -1.5±10 ml. The magnitude of the difference in volume measurement between 3DE and cine-ventriculography was significantly smaller using the Doppler technique for both end-diastole and end-systole.

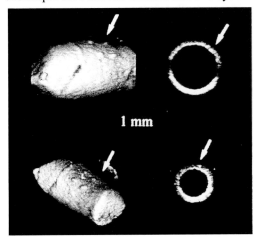

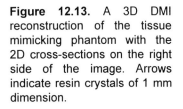

Figure 12.13. A 3D DMI reconstruction of the tissue mimicking phantom with the 2D cross-sections on the right side of the image. Arrows indicate resin crystals of 1 mm dimension.

To determine whether transthoracic 3DE could accurately define atrial septal defect (AS) morphology (Figure 12.14), 30 ASD patients were studied [28]. In each patient, two techniques were used to acquire 3D data: GSI and DMI. 3D images were constructed to simulate the surgeons view of the ASD (Figure 12.15). Measured parameters were maximum and minimum vertical (V) and horizontal (H) ASD dimension (D), distances to inferior (IVC) and superior vena cava (SVC), coronary sinus (CS), tricuspid valve (TV) (Figure 12.16). The maximum ASD D's were compared with magnetic resonance phase-contrast cine imaging (MRI) and surgery [28] (Table 12.1). In small children, measurement feasibility was similar for both techniques but higher for DMI than GSI in adult ASD patients (age > 17 years): maximum D 100% vs 81% min. D 91% vs 73%, SVC 82% vs 64%, IVC 82% vs 73%, CS 81% vs 55%, TV 100% vs 82%; respectively. Both DMI and GSI images showed dynamic change in ASD size during the cardiac cycle. Good correlation was found between 3DE and both MRI (DMI & GSI; 0.97) and surgery (DMI & GSI; 0.91) [3] (Figure 12.17). The bias between 3DE and (1) MRI: DMI=2.6 mm, GSI=3.4 mm (Figure 12.18), and (2) surgery: DMI=5 mm, GSI=5.6 mm (Figure 12.19). This study has shown that 3DE accurately displays the varying morphology, size and spatial relationships of an ASD. As a DMI data set it provides the optimum information on which to base patient management decisions.

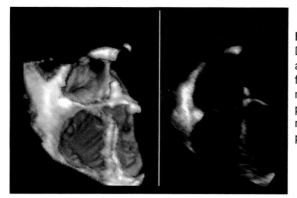

Figure 12.14. A 3D DMI reconstruction of an ASD seen from the four chamber view. The right part of the image presents the corresponding 2D cutplane.

Doppler Imaging of Skeletal Mode

Potential applications of DMI are not confined to cardiac imaging. Early validation work has demonstrated that DMI could be used to identify contracting skeletal muscle groups. Since then, a systematic examination of skeletal muscle contraction in healthy volunteers has been undertaken [29]. This study demonstrated the capability of DMI to identify tetanic skeletal muscle contraction, to differentiate between active contraction and passive muscle movement, and to characterize isotonic, isometric and reflex skeletal muscle contraction profiles. Thus, there may be considerable potential for further evaluation of DMI in neurological and musculoskeletal applications. In particular, DMI may have practical applications in the design and validation of biomechanical assist systems such as latissimus dorsi cardiomyoplasty [30.31].

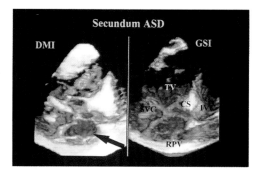

Figure 12.15. A 3D reconstruction of an ASD as seen by the surgeon. The left part of the image presents DMI information, the right part presents the GSI information. CS - coronary sinus, IVC - vena cava inferior, SVC - vena cava superior, TV - tricuspid valve, RPV - right pulmonary veins

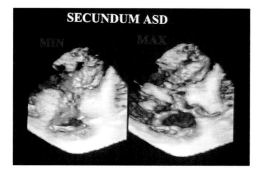

Figure 12.16. A 3D DMI reconstruction of the surgical view of an ASD demonstrating the changes in its size during the cardiac cycle.

Conclusions

DMI is a valuable addition to the clinical ultrasound investigative modalities providing new information not available from current standard echo techniques. The possible areas of clinical use of aspects of the technique are shown in Figure 12.20. At present, it remains a technique in its early stages of development. However, with sufficient frame-rates, resolution improvement, the development of off-line angle-independent velocity estimation and the implementation of multiple pulsed Doppler sample volumes its diagnostic range should be further extended.

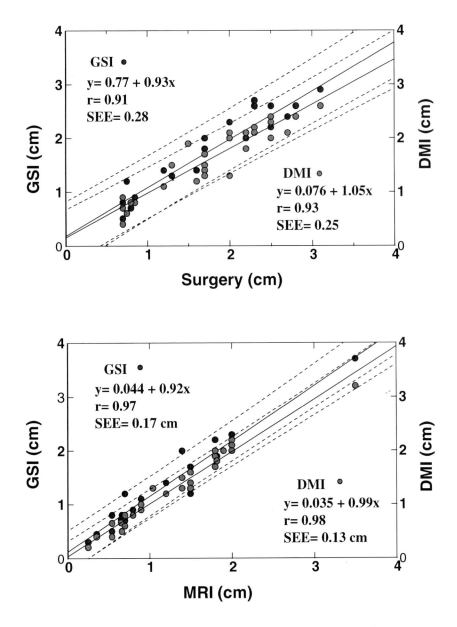

Figure 12.17. ASD measurements by 3D echocardiography against: surgery (top), and MRI (bottom).

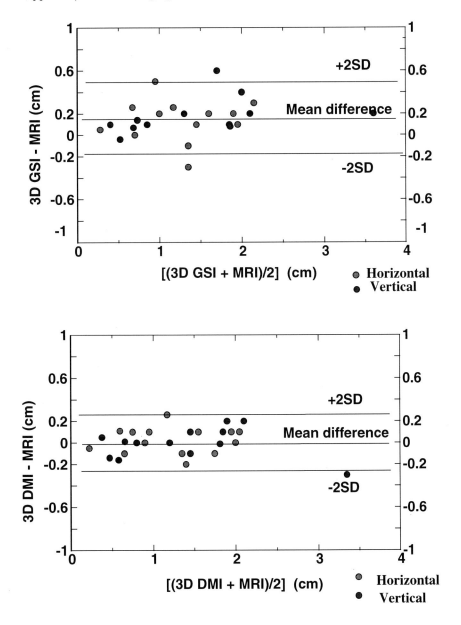

Figure 12.18. Differences between 3D GSI (top) and 3D DMI (bottom) versus MRI in ASD sizing.

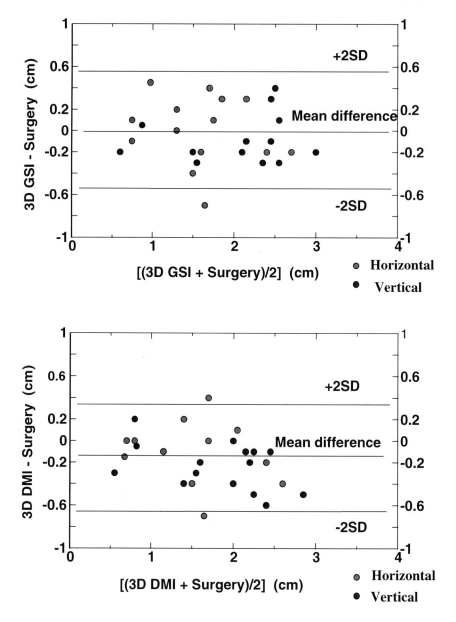

Figure 12.19. Differences between 3D GSI (top) and 3D DMI (bottom) versus surgery in ASD sizing.

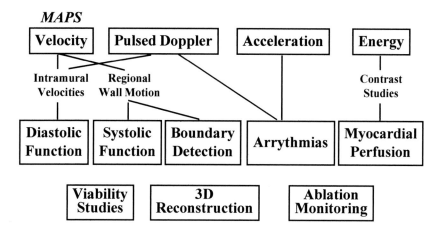

Figure 12.20. The potential clinical roles of Doppler myocardial imaging.

Comparison of ASD measurements taken from 3D images				
	Maximum		Minimum	
(cm)	HD	VD	HD	VD
GSI	1.9 ±0.8*	1.5 ±0.6*	1.3 ±0.8	0.9 ±0.5
DMI	1.7 ±0.7*	1.5 ±0.6*	1.2 ±0.7	0.9 ±0.5

*, compared to minimum, p< 0.01, by ANOVA

ASD, Atrial Septal Defect; DMI, Doppler Myocardial Imaging;
GSI, Grey-Scale Imaging; HD, Horizontal ASD Dimension;
VD, Vertical ASD Dimension

Table 12.1. Comparison of ASD measurements taken from 3D images.

References

1. Sutherland GR, Stewart J, Grounstroem KWE, Moran CM, Fleming AD, Guell-Peris PJ, Riemersma RA, Fenn LN, Fox KAA, McDicken WN: Color Doppler myocardial imaging: A new technique for the assessment of myocardial function. *J Am Soc Echocardiogr* 1994;7:441-458.

2. Miyatake K, Yamagishi M, Tanaka N, Uematsu M, Vamazaki N, Mine V, Sano A: A new method for the evaluation of left ventricular wall motion by color-coded tissue Doppler imaging: *In vitro* and *in vivo* studies. *J Am Coll Cardiol* *1995;25:717-724.*

3. Issaz K, Thomson A, Ethevenot G, Cloez JL, Brembella B, Pernot C: Doppler echocardiographic measurement of low velocity motion of the left ventricular posterior wall. *Am J Cardiol* 1989;64:66-75.

4. McDicken WN, Sutherland GR, Moran CM, Gordon L: Color Doppler velocity imaging of the myocardium. *Ultrasound Med Biol* 1992;18:651-654.

5. Fleming AD, McDicken WN, Sutherland GR, Hoskins PR: Assessment of color Doppler tissue imaging using test phantoms. *Ultrasound Med Biol* 1994;20:937-51.

6. Schwarz KQ, Bezante GP, Chen X. When can Doppler be used in place of integrated backscatter as a measure of scattered ultrasound intensity? *Ultrasound Med Biol* 1995;21:231-242.

7. Fleming AD, Xia X, McDicken WN, Sutherland GR, Fenn L: Myocardial velocity gradient by Doppler imaging. *Br J Radiol* 1994;67:679-688.

8. Fleming AD, Palka P, McDicken WN, Sutherland GR: Verification of cardiac Doppler tissue images using grey-scale M-Mode images. *Ultrasound Med Biol* 1996;22 (in press).

9. Palka P, Lange A, Fleming AD, Sutherland GR, Fenn LN, McDicken WN: Doppler tissue imaging: Myocardial wall motion abnormalities in normal subjects. *J Am Soc Echocardiogr* 1995;8:659-668.

10. Palka P, Fleming AD, Lange A, Fenn LN, Sutherland GR, McDicken WN: Doppler myocardial imaging: Mean myocardial velocity and velocity gradient in normal subjects. *Br Heart J* 1996;73:85 (Abstract).

11. Rodriguez L, Garcia M, Ares M, Leung D, Thomas JD, Griffin B: Is mitral annulus motion during early diastole active or passive? Clinical evidence of elastic recoil. *J Am Coll Cardiol* 1995;25:P57A (Abstract).

12. Rodriguez L, Garcia M, Nakatani S, Ares M, Griffin B, Thomas JD: Longitudinal axis diastolic dynamics in patients with left ventricular hypertrophy: A Doppler tissue imaging study. *J Am Soc Echocardiogr* 1995;8:391 (Abstract).

13. Rodriguez L, Garcia M, Nakatani S, Leung D, Grimm R, Griffin B, Thomas JD: Quantitation of left atrial systolic function by Doppler tissue imaging: Clinical validation. *J Am Soc Echocardiogr* 1995;8:349 (Abstract).

14. Rodriguez L, Nakatani S, Leung D, Griffin B, Stewart W, Thomas JD, Grimm R: Measurement of atrial appendage cycle length by transthoracic echocardiography using Doppler tissue imaging. *J Am Soc Echocardiogr* 1995;8:391 (Abstract).

15. Lange A, Palka P, Sutherland GR, Fleming AD, Fenn LN, Bouki KP, Wright RA, Ramo P, McDicken WN: Doppler tissue imaging assessment of systolic and diastolic transmural velocity gradients in dilated cardiomyopathy: A new diagnostic index. *Eur Heart J* 1995;16:298 (Abstract).

16. Palka P, Lange A, Sutherland GR, Fleming AD, Fenn LN, Bouki K, Ramo P, McDicken WN: Doppler tissue imaging: Assessment of systolic and diastolic

transmural velocity gradients in hypertrophic cardiomyopathy. A new diagnostic index. *Eur Heart J* 1995;16:105 (Abstract).

17. Uematsu M, Miyatake K, Tanaka N, Matsuda H, Sano A, Yamazaki N, Hirama M, Yamagishi M: Myocardial velocity gradient as a new indicator of regional left ventricular contraction: Detection by a two dimensional tissue Doppler imaging technique. *J Am Coll Cardiol* 1995;26:217-223.

18. Stewart MJ, Sutherland GR, Moran CN, Fleming AD, Fenn LN, McDicken WN: Imaging of ischemic and infarcted myocardium by Doppler tissue imaging. *Circulation* 1993;88:1-47 (Abstract).

19. Garcia-Fernandez MA, Azevedo J, Puerta M, Moreno E, Torrecilla E, San Roman D: Quantitative analysis of segmental left ventricular wall dysfunction by pulsed Doppler tissue imaging: A new insight into diastolic performance. *Eur Heart J* 1995;16:451 (Abstract).

20. von Bibra H, Tuchnitz A, Firschke C, Schohlen H, Schomig A: Doppler tissue imaging of left ventricular myocardium - initial results during pharmacologic stress. *J Am Coll Cardiol* 1995;25:P57A (Abstract).

21. Fontanet HL, Puleo JA, Davis MG, Lockely M: Quantitative dobutamine stress echocardiography utilizing Doppler tissue imaging. *J Am Coll Cardiol* 1996;27:65A (Abstract).

22. Sutherland GR, von Bibra H, Tuchnitz A, Henke J, Schonig A: Transthoracic detection of regional myocardial perfusion abnormalities using a pervenous contrast agent - A comparative study of Doppler energy and grey scale imaging. *Br Heart J* 1995;73:57 (Abstract).

23. Yamagishi M, Tanaka N, Itoh S, Miyatake K, Yamayahi N, Hirama M: An enhanced method for detection of early contraction site of ventricles in Wolff-Parkinson-White syndrome using color coded tissue Doppler echocardiography. *J Am Soc Echocardiogr* 1993;6:30 (Abstract).

24. Sutherland GR, Pons Llado GP, Carreras F, Vinolas X, Oter R, Subiren M, Bayes de Luna: Doppler myocardial imaging in the evaluation of normal and abnormal ventricular depolarization. *Br Heart J* 1995;73:85 (Abstract).

25. Lange A, Palka P, Caso P, Fenn LN, Olszewski R, Ramo MP, Shaw TRD, Nowicki A, Fox KAA, Sutherland GR: Doppler myocardial imaging versus B-Mode grey-scale imaging: A comparative *in vitro* and *in vivo* study into their relative efficacy in endocardial boundary detection. *Ultrasound Med Biol* (in press).

26. Sutherland GR, Caso P, Palka P, Fenn LN, Lange A, McDicken WN: Doppler myocardial imaging assessment of left ventricular volume and area - a comparison with grey-scale imaging. *Eur Heart J* 1995;16:392 (Abstract).

27. Lange A, Bouki K, Fenn LN, Palka P, McDicken WN, Sutherland WN: A comparison study of grey scale versus Doppler tissue imaging left ventricular volume measurement using three dimensional reconstruction. *Eur Heart J* 1995;16:266 (Abstract).

28. Lange A, Palka P, Sutherland GR, Shaw TRD, Fox KAA, Godman MJ: Three-dimensional definition of dynamic atrial septal defect morphology by transthoracic echocardiography. *Eur Heart J* 1996;17:425 (Abstract).

29. Grubb NR, Fleming A, Fox KAA, Sutherland GR: Evaluation of Doppler tissue imaging for the assessment of skeletal muscle function in healthy volunteers. *Radiology* 1995;194:837-842.

30. Grubb NR, Sutherland GR, Campanella C: Optimization of myostimulation dynamic cardiomyoplasty. *Eur J Cardiothoracic Surg* 1995;9:45-49.

31. Grubb NR, Sutherland GR, Campanella C, Fleming A, Sinclair C Fox KAA: Latissimus dorsi muscle: Assessment of stimulation after cardiomyopathy with Doppler ultrasound tissue imaging. Radiology 1996;199:59-64.

INDEX

Note: Page numbers in italics refer to figures; page numbers followed by *t* indicate tables.